# England vs Scotland

## Does More Money Mean Better Health?

Benedict Irvine
Ian Ginsberg

Commentary
Kevin Woods

Civitas: Institute for the Study of Civil Society
London

First published June 2004

© The Institute for the Study of Civil Society 2004
77 Great Peter Street
London SW1P 2EZ
email: books@civitas.org.uk

ISBN 1-903 386-35-7

Typeset by Civitas
in New Century Schoolbook

Printed in Great Britain by
Hartington Fine Arts,
Lancing, Sussex

# Contents

# *Authors*

**Ian Ginsberg** graduated with a first from Trinity Hall Cambridge, where he also completed a Masters. He joined Civitas as a full-time researcher in 2002. He now works in the public health and performance directorate for a strategic health authority.

**Benedict Irvine** is director of the Civitas Health Unit. After studying law he completed a Master's degree in comparative European public administration at the Catholic University of Leuven, Belgium. Before joining Civitas he worked as a researcher in the European Parliament. He has managed a wide range of comparative projects on European healthcare funding and provision. Recent work has included a study of the relationship between healthcare funding systems and health outcomes. Current projects include an examination of the pricing and reimbursement of pharmaceuticals in Europe. He is also secretary to the cross-spectrum UK Health Care Consensus Group.

**Kevin Woods** has held a number of general management positions in the NHS in England. He was appointed to the Lindsay Chair of Health Policy and Economic Evaluation, University of Glasgow in August 2000. He established the Scottish Health Services Policy Forum, which promotes debate about health services in post-devolution Scotland. Previously he was director of strategy and performance management for the NHS in Scotland working with the Scottish Office (now Scottish Executive) Department of Health. In January 2004 he returned to the NHS in England. He has published on Scotland's health and health services, social deprivation, resource allocation and healthcare planning. Ongoing research interests include health system integration and healthcare rationing.

# *Acknowledgements*

This project was sponsored by Andrew Ferguson on behalf of the David Hume Institute. Staff at the ISD in Scotland and the NHS National Cancer Services Analysis Team in England were helpful. We would like also to acknowledge the vital comparative work of the OECD Health Team, and the devolution monitoring and analysis of the Constitution Unit based at UCL. The staff of the King's Fund library were as helpful as ever. Further thanks should go to two referees for their helpful comments on an earlier draft of this report.

# Preface

The purpose of this research exercise was to examine the thesis, propounded by the Blair Government in England, that the widely acknowledged problems and deficiencies of the NHS can be resolved by substantially increasing expenditure.

Using the example of Scotland, where health expenditure per head already approaches the European average to which the Government aspires, we explore whether (with due allowance for any 'Scottish effect') increased expenditure has produced better health care for patients.

We collated data on expenditure, treatment resources, activity rates, population and environmental inputs, the use of standard treatments, and healthcare outcomes. In light of this evidence, albeit with caveats regarding data quality and comparability, we find the case 'not proven'. On this assumption, we further conclude that additional reform is likely to be necessary to deliver the improvements desired by patients, healthcare professionals and politicians. Perhaps structural change of healthcare funding is a necessary condition? And if the extra per capita spending in Scotland had been from another funding source, would outcomes have improved?

The funding and provision of health care is a thorny issue because of the dual character of medical demand. On the one hand, severe pain or dysfunction may prevent people from leading a normal life, and in extreme cases life or death may be at stake. On the other hand, some demands for medical services are a matter of personal preference. No less important, some ill health is a matter of sheer misfortune and some a consequence of harmful lifestyle choices.

Public policy makers continue to struggle with these conundrums in all countries, but I conclude that some have devised solutions which have proved more effective than others. In particular, countries with social insurance systems (Germany, France, the Netherlands and Switzerland) have the most to teach us.[1] So are our political leaders willing to learn from these alternatives?

In England, there has been a palpable shift; it is now possible seriously to raise questions about the NHS that would have been condemned as heretical only a few years ago. In October 2003, a King's Fund report suggested that politicians should be taken out of the management of healthcare.[2] In November 2003, LSE Health published a report showing that access to healthcare is better for the middle classes—who know how to 'play' the NHS system.[3] Such reports illustrate a shift in the terms of the debate and in the latter case suggest that the myth of health care based on need, not ability to pay, is just that—a myth. The shift in the debate is especially noted by those working in the English NHS. Meanwhile, after 50 years of comparatively poor performance from the NHS in Scotland, it is surprising that (other than for clinical lessons), unlike their counterparts in all political parties in England, Scots decision-makers do not appear to have made a concerted effort to learn from foreign healthcare systems. Yes, there are other state-run quasi-monopoly systems that seem to work better, most notably that in Sweden, though of course it is local government that is in the revenue-raising and management driving seat there, making for a much more transparent system. Nevertheless, bearing in mind evidence from the OECD, there is a compelling case for both Scots and the English to call for more radical reform of the NHS; ideally through the introduction of competitive social insurance—perhaps the most important element of which is the removal of national politicians from the day-to-day running of the system. Such a move may lead in time to long-overdue improvement in Scottish and English health outcomes relative to our neighbours.

## A solution?

Civitas has studied healthcare systems in Europe and further afield. We take it as axiomatic that the basic building block of any reform must be ready access for all patients to a government-guaranteed high standard of care. Every country is wrestling with how to achieve this end and many have discovered alternative methods which have secured a more responsive and demonstrably higher quality service than that provided through the NHS. While none provide a ready-made blueprint, we should be willing to learn from their experiences.[4] We propose the following:[5]

- The primary role of government should be to create the legal and regulatory framework, to ensure that access to a high standard of care is guaranteed to all, and to ensure the supply of essential public health services.

- Politicians should be excluded from management of healthcare. They must not override the professional duty of clinicians to act in the interests of patients.

- The responsibility for financing health care should be divorced from the responsibility to supply.

- Health insurance should be compulsory and patients should be free to choose from among a range of third-party payers.

- There should be no compulsory patient charges at point of use—though they might be optional.

- Health care should be provided by competing healthcare organisations (including for-profit companies, charities or non-profit trusts), thus enabling the efficiencies in supply provided by competing suppliers and allowing consumer choice.

- A new 'information agency' would be useful to monitor standards and provide impartial statistical comparisons allowing effective choice based on outcome and real measurement of trends.[6]

- The Government should not own hospitals and all such institutions currently in the public sector should become independent at the earliest possible date. The simplest method would be to make them all foundation hospitals, whilst ensuring that their assets must be permanently used to provide health care. Existing NHS hospitals should not be transferred to the ownership of for-profit institutions.

- Hospitals should have complete autonomy from White-
  hall and the Scottish Executive. In particular, there
  should be no specific restrictions (beyond those that apply
  to all workplaces) on the ability of hospitals to recruit
  staff or on the conditions of their employment.

- The Government has an important role in ensuring that
  hospital accident and emergency infrastructure is
  universally available. In the rare event of a hospital
  being in financial difficulty, the Government must be able
  to take appropriate action.

- There should be no restrictions on the establishment of
  new hospitals, whether they are for-profit or not, as at
  present.

As Kevin Woods (Lindsay Professor of Health Policy and
Economic Evaluation at the University of Glasgow) suggests
in his commentary, if this paper helps to facilitate an
informed debate on reforming the NHS in Scotland and
England, it will be worthwhile. Of course, as for most
comparative research, our findings are subject to numerous
caveats regarding the quality and comparability of data,
differences between sexes and regions, and the different
provider structures in England and Scotland. Nevertheless
some trends are clear. It is to be expected that there will be
discussions about the quality of our data and their comparability. But the danger is that those reading this report seize
upon the minutiae of international comparisons and remain
in their well-established pro-NHS and anti-NHS positions
without engaging in a long-overdue debate about systems
that fail patients daily.

Finally, readers should note that this report reflects the
data that were available and structures as they were in
spring and early summer of 2003. There have been important changes and new data sources since then. And further
relevant data are due, including a new EUROCARE III
study. More resources are being dedicated to heart disease
and cancer care. More specialist technology is being purchased in England and Scotland. And healthcare structures
are continually evolving—arguably in different directions

north and south of the border. We see greater choice and competition on the supply-side in England, while healthcare is becoming more integrated in Scotland. The Civitas website publishes an up-to-date review of the literature on whether the extra spending on the NHS in England is having the desired effect.

http://www.civitas.org.uk/nhs/nhsMoney.php

*Benedict Irvine*

# *Summary*

We know that health systems subject to central political management tend to limit the availability of resources, especially the number of doctors, in the belief that medical demand is 'supplier induced' and has little bearing on medical outcomes. However, more recent research shows that there is an optimal spending level that varies over time, typically increasing with per capita income. Higher total expenditure on health than in the UK and a higher number of doctors per head than in the UK are both correlated to improved medical outcomes. Jeremy Hurst of the OECD concludes:

> The evidence on both health outcomes and waiting times suggests, if only superficially, that *countries tend to get what they pay for.* Premature mortality declines as physician numbers increase and waiting times for specialist care decline as expenditure per capita rises'.[1]

But Scotland may be an exception to the rule.

- Total expenditure on healthcare per capita is correlated with health status.[2] Increased expenditure leads to improved health outcomes.[3] A cluster of consistently higher indicators is found among those countries spending $1,700 purchasing power parity (PPP) per capita, or more. Beyond that threshold, one does not find a clear positive correlation between performance and increased expenditure.[4]

- The availability of medical resources has a beneficial impact on medical outcomes. The number of doctors per head affects medical outcomes. Infant and maternal mortality are significantly reduced when the number of physicians increases.[5] Avoidable mortality, when medical intervention is capable of having an impact, also improves with the number of doctors.[6] For some reason, Scotland's superior levels of healthcare resources do not lead to generally better health outcomes.

- More frequent use of accepted medical technologies is associated with improved outcomes. For example, the use of specialist units in the treatment of stroke patients is strongly correlated with improved outcomes. Specialist units are under-used in the UK.[7] The rate of CABG and PTCA vary significantly between countries. Both Scotland and England lag behind, arguably for financial reasons.[8]

Of course great caution must be taken when comparing healthcare systems and drawing conclusions from those comparisons. Nevertheless, the common observation that Scotland already spends the EU average of its GDP on health care, but does not deliver 'average' levels of health, may suggest that the organisation of the healthcare system is a key explanation. Of course Scotland, like England, has a state-run as well as a funded system rather than a social-insurance system with multiple non-government actors. However, there are competing hypotheses, notably the view that social deprivation is more prevalent in Scotland.

Despite this latter view, it is our contention, that without further reform, the Government's pledge to raise health spending in England to the EU levels may only mimic the experience in Scotland, whereby increased spending appears to result in higher costs of production rather than better outcomes or more responsive services.

# Introduction

## Objectives

Healthcare responsibilities are devolved to the four constituent countries of the UK: Northern Ireland, Wales, Scotland and England. The objective of this report is to make an assessment of the funding, quality and performance of NHS health services in England and Scotland. Our main aim is to explore the hypothesis that increasing healthcare expenditure in England may not yield improvements in patient care sufficient to raise England to the standards found in other countries such as Switzerland and France; Scotland already spends at the higher level to which England aspires without achieving French/Swiss standards.

### Setting the scene

The latest publication of the OECD's health data has again shown the poor quality of UK healthcare compared to other countries.[1] The statistics show that victims of heart disease, stroke or breast cancer in Britain die early, and perhaps unnecessarily, compared with most other western countries. Worse still, it seems that access to care is being limited according to age. Roger Dobson, a regular contributor to the *British Medical Journal*, reports on an international study that found the proportion of health spending on those aged 65+ in England and Wales is not keeping track with that in other countries.[2] Dr Alastair Gray and Meena Seshamani from the Health Economics Research Centre at Oxford University found:

> In contrast to the findings of previous studies, this analysis of health expenditure data has found that in England and Wales the high cost older groups did not have larger increases in their medical costs than the middle age-groups. In fact ... the oldest old had decreases in their real per capita costs, while other age-groups experienced real cost increases.[3]

1

*) e*
*does not*
*follow*

The same researchers noted that data from the OECD show that in developed countries per capita spending for those aged over 65 has increased at the same rate or faster than among those aged under 65. The UK bucks this trend.

Do these findings suggest that the NHS in England (and perhaps Scotland) suffers from a systemic flaw that can only be overcome by radical change? Have other systems proved better able to avoid rationing by keeping the resources available for treatment in balance with medical demand?[4]

## Methodology

Health system analysis is complex. We have used an inputs and outputs model as our analytical framework. In the healthcare context, inputs can be narrowed down to the health of the population, and the financial resources dedicated to it. Meanwhile, outputs are synonymous with health outcome (see figure 1, p. 5).[5] Intermediate healthcare outcomes, that is those which follow healthcare system processes (e.g. doctor-patient contact), can be positive or negative and can indicate quality of health care. These 'healthcare outcomes' are distinguished from 'health outcome', which is determined by important factors in addition to the health system, such as population structure, education, degree of deprivation, environment and so forth.[6]

We use this framework as a guide, however certain elements of it lie outside the scope of this report, namely the environment, other systems, and the education system. Nevertheless, these elements are borne in mind during our later discussion.

There were two main methods of inquiry: a literature review covering longitudinal and comparative published and other literature over the past 20 years and more; and the identification and assessment of routine health inputs and outcomes data that might provide insights into our main research question.

Comparing systems is notoriously controversial, some thinking it an important source of inspiration, while others consider the exercise a complete waste of time.[7] It is generally accepted that healthcare arrangements in one country cannot be transplanted into another owing to historical, cultural and political differences, nevertheless we strongly believe that there are important lessons to be learned by comparing healthcare systems. It is thought that healthcare systems have at best only a minimal impact (c. ten per cent) on the health of a population. However, this well-established received wisdom is being increasingly challenged as studies have shown that the presence of effective health care available when it is needed (avoidable mortality) leads to declining mortality.[8]

There are numerous methodological difficulties when carrying out comparative research. It is necessary to approach data collection and analysis with caution in order to guarantee that like is compared with like. Socio-economic deprivation has been at the centre of much analysis of Scotland's health outcomes.[9] Carstairs' work which examines the extent to which differences in deprivation levels between Scotland, England and Wales, explain differences in mortality, being most famous.[10] Carstairs showed that a larger proportion of the Scottish population lives in the most deprived areas. Perhaps because of our reliance on published material, we encountered some difficulty in the course of this project, particularly with regard to the population standardisation for cancer and heart disease data. The lack of standardisation between regions and countries of recording/registration of activity and outcomes also presented problems. These difficulties are only highlighted by the fact that the international agencies collecting widely cited comparable health data such as the OECD, WHO and Eurostat, often do not include specific Scottish data. The EUROCARE study offers an exception to this trend, however the EUROCARE findings regarding incidence and survival are also described as an artefact because Scottish data registration is unusually complete; perhaps making Scotland appear comparatively worse than it really is. Problems apply for cardiovascular disease comparisons too: 'International comparisons of Scottish cardiovascular mortality and morbidity rely heavily on data collected in the

Glasgow arm of the MONICA study which though of high quality, is not representative of Scotland as a whole'.[11] Finally, when comparing Scotland with England, it is important to note that the English population is nearly ten times the size of the Scottish population and that Scotland covers a smaller and more rural area of land than the England. Both factors have some bearing on the operation of the healthcare system.[12] Cautionary notes on data sources are included where appropriate.

We start by looking at the inputs to the Scottish and English health systems, that is, financial resources and the demographic structure and health inputs of the population. This is followed by comparison of patient benefits. Then we briefly look at health system resources and organisation. The majority remainder of the report presents health outcomes and some treatment processes information. A short discussion of our findings precedes a commentary by Professor Kevin Woods, Lindsay Professor of Health Policy and Economic Evaluation at the University of Glasgow.

5

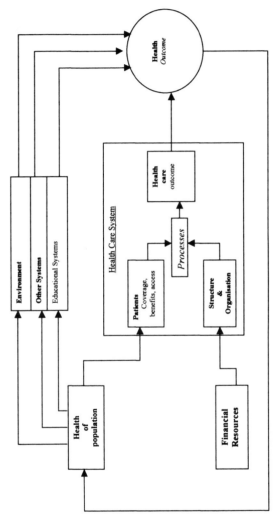

*Figure 1*
*Health Inputs-Outputs Model*

Source: reproduced from Busse, R, *Health Care Systems: Britain and Germany Compared*, Anglo-German Foundation for the Study of Industrial Society, 2002.

# 1

# Healthcare Funding and Expenditure

- Healthcare expenditure
- Main system of funding
- Private medical funding
- Healthcare resource distribution
- Risk adjustment

*Expenditure in NHS England and Scotland*[1]

Over the past 20 years, total healthcare expenditure as a percentage of GDP in the UK has remained 1-1.5 per cent below the EU average, and even further behind major competitors France and Germany.[2] Total national health-care expenditure characteristics in the UK and a number of other countries are presented in Table 1.1.[3] In 2002, the NHS cost the average British household £2,400 per year. That is roughly £1,000 per person. But if we examine the data in more detail, we find that per capita spending on health and personal social services in 2000-2001 was higher in Scotland (£1,347) than England (£1,132) and the UK average (£1,163) (see Table 1.2).[4] Health spending in Scotland is equivalent to 116 per cent of UK and 119 per cent of English spending.[5] Scotland also spends more in GDP terms; in July 2000, Susan Deacon, the Scottish health minister, announced 'that in 1997 public expenditure on health in Scotland amounted to 6.4 per cent of its GDP, compared with the EU average of 6.5 per cent and a UK average of 5.8 per cent'.[6] Table 1.1 indicates that these figures are now out of date, but the trends between England, Scotland and the EU remain valid.

6

## Table 1.1
### Expenditure characteristics, latest available figures (LAF)

| Characteristic | France | Germany | UK | EU | USA |
|---|---|---|---|---|---|
| US$PPP-econ-wide per capita | 2,349 | 2,451 (98) | 1,763 (99) | 1,937 | 4,358 (99) 1 |
| Main £ source | SI | SI | Tax | Tax/SI | PI/Tax |
| % public £ / TEH and 1990-8 trends | 76 +/- | 75.8 (98) +/- | 81.0 - | 74.4 (98) | 44.5 (99) ++ |
| % GDP (2000) OECD + EU (8.0) | 9.5 | 10.6 | 7.3 | 8.0 | 13.0 |
| % GDP rank | 3 | 2 | 5 | 4 | 1 |

*Source*: OECD Health Data 2002. Unless otherwise indicated (99), figures given are from 2000. EU averages are those for all 15 member countries, with the exception of US$PPP-econ-wide, where Sweden, Luxembourg and Germany are excluded as data are not available.
*Note*: SI = social insurance; PI = private insurance.

## Table 1.2
### Identifiable total managed public expenditure by country

**Identifiable total managed expenditure, by country, £m**

| | 1996-97 | 1997-98 | 1998-99 | 1999-00 | 2000-01 |
|---|---|---|---|---|---|
| England | 193,280 | 196,336 | 202,288 | 213,044 | 226,446 |
| Scotland | 24,680 | 25,029 | 25,830 | 26,970 | 28,428 |
| UK | 240,719 | 244,464 | 252,155 | 264,924 | 281,402 |

**Identifiable total managed expenditure, as a percentage of UK total**

| | 1996-97 (%) | 1997-98 (%) | 1998-99 (%) | 1999-00 (%) | 2000-01 (%) |
|---|---|---|---|---|---|
| England | 80.29 | 80.31 | 80.22 | 80.42 | 80.47 |
| Scotland | 10.25 | 10.24 | 10.24 | 10.18 | 10.10 |
| UK | 100.00 | 100.00 | 100.00 | 100.00 | 100.00 |

**Identifiable total managed expenditure, per head by country, £per head**

| | 1996-97 | 1997-98 | 1998-99 | 1999-00 | 2000-01 |
|---|---|---|---|---|---|
| England | 3,937 | 3,984 | 4,087 | 4,282 | 4,529 |
| Scotland | 4,813 | 4,886 | 5,045 | 5,268 | 5,558 |
| UK | 4,093 | 4,142 | 4,257 | 4,452 | 4,709 |

**Identifiable total managed expenditure, per head by country, relative to UK**

| | 1996-97 | 1997-98 | 1998-99 | 1999-00 | 2000-01 |
|---|---|---|---|---|---|
| England | 96 | 96 | 96 | 96 | 96 |
| Scotland | 118 | 118 | 119 | 118 | 118 |

*Source*: Public Expenditure Statistical Analyses 2002-2003, Chapter 8.

## Table 1.3
### Identifiable public expenditure on health by country

**Identifiable expenditure on health, by country, £m**

|          | 1996-97 | 1997-98 | 1998-99 | 1999-00 | 2000-01 |
|----------|---------|---------|---------|---------|---------|
| England  | 42,733  | 44,894  | 47,634  | 51,804  | 56,583  |
| Scotland | 5,610   | 5,751   | 6,017   | 6,473   | 6,888   |
| UK       | 52,961  | 55,482  | 58,753  | 63,771  | 69,489  |

**Identifiable expenditure on health, by country, £per head**

|          | 1996-97 | 1997-98 | 1998-99 | 1999-00 | 2000-01 |
|----------|---------|---------|---------|---------|---------|
| England  | 871     | 911     | 962     | 1,041   | 1,132   |
| Scotland | 1,094   | 1,123   | 1,175   | 1,264   | 1,347   |
| UK       | 901     | 940     | 992     | 1,072   | 1,163   |

**Identifiable expenditure on health, by country as a percentage of UK total**

|          | 1996-97 | 1997-98 | 1998-99 | 1999-00 | 2000-01 |
|----------|---------|---------|---------|---------|---------|
| England  | 81      | 81      | 81      | 81      | 81      |
| Scotland | 11      | 10      | 10      | 10      | 10      |
| UK       | 100     | 100     | 100     | 100     | 100     |

*Source*: Public Expenditure Statistical Analyses 2002-2003, Chapter 8.

Public spending levels in England and Scotland are set by the UK Comprehensive Spending Review (CSR), on a three-yearly cycle. The division of total managed expenditure between Scotland and England has remained stable over recent years (see Table 1.2). England spends just over 80 per cent of the UK total (c. £226 billion), while Scotland spends fractionally over 10 per cent (c. £28 billion). Expenditure on the NHS in Scotland each year is decided upon by the first minister for Scotland within the overall resources available to him following the CSR. In 1998-99, a third of the Scottish Executive budget was spent on the health service—this amounted to some £4.97 billion.[7] Table 1.3 shows identifiable public expenditure on health in England and Scotland.

There are a number of issues to note with regard to healthcare funding in Scotland. Funding for the Scottish health department comes from the Scottish 'block' of UK public spending, as formulated by the UK government's triennial public expenditure survey. The Barnett formula is then applied to any increases or decreases to departmental expenditure levels in England to give the proportionate increase or decrease in the devolved countries' spending.[8] The formula does theoretically allow for a disproportionate increase in the healthcare allocation in Scotland, as the Scottish Executive has discretionary powers to use the extra money allocated to it in any way it sees fit. For example, an increase in social care spending in England will generate an increase in the overall Scottish 'block', and this can be used for health.[9] Table 1.3 above shows that there has been stability between Scotland and England in the division of identifiable expenditure on health as a percentage of UK total.

Amid consensus that the NHS has been underfunded for many years, both countries have seen recent rises in public healthcare expenditure. In 2000, the Scottish health budget increased by an extra £481 million, taking the total budget to c. £5.5 billion. The budget was due to rise to £6.7 billion in 2003-04, but subsequent promises mean this sum was achieved by 2002-2003.[10] Following the review and recommendations by Derek Wanless, expenditure on the NHS in England is also set to rise in the next few years.[11] In his spring budget 2002, the Chancellor of the Exchequer announced a 7.4 per cent (real terms) per year increase in public spending on the NHS between 2002-03 and 2007-08.[12] Over this period the UK NHS budget is set to rise by over 44 per cent in real terms to over £90 billion in 2007-08.[13] Table 1.4 below shows increasing levels of NHS spending. Though we have seen that spending per capita in Scotland has been higher than England for some time, recent and future increases will see the relative position of England improve.[14]

**Table 1.4**
*Public healthcare budgets in England and Scotland*

|          | 2000-2001 | 2001-2002 | 2002-2003 | 2003-2004 |
|----------|-----------|-----------|-----------|-----------|
| Scotland | £5.5 bn   | £6.2 bn   | £6.7 bn   | £7.1 bn   |
| England  | £44.2 bn  | £48.0 bn  | £52.0 bn  | £56.4 bn  |
| UK       | £54.2 bn  | £58.6 bn  | £63.5 bn  | £69.7 bn  |

*Sources*: Scotland: 'Health and Community Care - The Scottish Budget 2003-2004'. England: Wellard's 2001-02; Public Expenditure Statistical Analyses 2002-2003.

As shown in Table 1.5, the Government Expenditure and Revenue in Scotland Report 2000-2001 identifies total managed expenditure in Scotland and the UK, by programme. Readers will note spending on health and personal social services is similar (24.2 per cent and 24.7 per cent respectively in Scotland and the UK [not England]) in terms of total public spending per programme.

*Components of NHS Expenditure*

In the UK in 2000, hospital and community health services and family health services discretionary spending (81 per cent of total NHS expenditure). The remaining 19 per cent was divided between capital spending (three per cent), family health services non-discretionary spending (GP remuneration, dental and ophthalmic services and pharmaceutical charges) (ten per cent), central; health services (public health) DOH administration (one per cent).[15] We do not have accurate data to differentiate between Scotland and England on NHS expenditure components.

**Funding Healthcare**

How much funding comes from taxes, social insurance, private insurance and out-of-pocket payment? What are the relative strengths of each?

Unlike the countries examined in our recent studies, which represent a cross section of the five funding arrangements found in advanced Western democracies,[16] Scotland and England are almost identical in their reliance on general taxation as a funding source. As public sector centralised systems they are found in the right hand column of Figure 1.1 (p. 12). Of course, no system is reliant on a sole source of finance. Rather, all systems rely on a mixture of public and private finance.[17] The balance between each of the many different forms of public and private funding sources varies and is constantly changing.[18] We have not found a detailed published breakdown of funding sources in England and Scotland. Rather, we use UK data and draw inferences from what we know about private insurance funding in Scotland and England.

11

## Table 1.5
### Identifiable total managed expenditure in Scotland and the UK, by programme, 2000-01

| Programme | Scotland Expenditure £m | Scotland Share of Identifiable Expenditure (%) | UK Expenditure £m | UK Share of Identifiable Expenditure (%) |
|---|---|---|---|---|
| Education | 4,747 | 16.7 | 44,628 | 15.9 |
| Health and Personal Social Services | 6,888 | 24.2 | 69,489 | 24.7 |
| Roads and transport | 947 | 3.3 | 9,002 | 3.2 |
| Housing | 469 | 1.6 | 3,347 | 1.2 |
| Other environmental services | 1,023 | 3.6 | 9,628 | 3.4 |
| Law, order and protective services | 1,806 | 6.4 | 20,239 | 7.2 |
| Trade, Industry, energy and employment | 1,000 | 3.5 | 7,571 | 2.7 |
| Agriculture, fisheries, food and forestry | 1,105 | 3.9 | 5,141 | 1.8 |
| Culture, media and sport | 429 | 1.5 | 5,529 | 2.0 |
| Social security | 9,816 | 34.5 | 103,853 | 36.9 |
| Miscellaneous expenditure | 196 | 0.7 | 2,974 | 1.1 |
| **Total** | 28,428 | 100.0 | 281,402 | 100.0 |

Source: Public Expenditure Statistical Analyses 2002-2003, Chapter 8.

## Figure 1.1
### Five types of healthcare financing schemes in Western Democracies

| Private model | Public models | | | |
| --- | --- | --- | --- | --- |
| Competitive insurance plans | Competitive insurance plans (a) | Employer-based insurance plans | Public sector: devolved | Public sector: centralised |
| USA 37* | Netherlands (b) 17 | France 1 | Denmark 34 | UK 18<br>Scotland (d)<br>England |
| Singapore 6 | Switzerland 20<br>Germany 25 | Netherlands (c) 17 | Canada 30<br>Spain 7 | |

*Source*: Based on Table 11.1, Rice, N and Smith P. 'Strategic resource allocation and funding decisions', in Mossialos, E., Dixon,*et al.*, 2002.

Notes:

* The numbers refer to the WHO 2000 overall ranking of each country's health system performance.

(a) Note German, Dutch and Belgian health insurance is employer based, while that in Switzerland is not.

(b) ZFW - Dutch second 'compartment'

(c) AWBZ - Dutch first 'compartment'

(d) Though healthcare is technically 'devolved', healthcare funding in Scotland is not akin to that in Scandinavian countries where much healthcare funding is raised locally.

## Table 1.6
## *Plurality and balance in healthcare finance in four countries*

| Country | Main source of finance | Public exp % TEH | Tax % TEH | Social Insurance % | Private exp % TEH | Voluntary Health Insurance | User Charges % TEH | Other % TEH |
|---|---|---|---|---|---|---|---|---|
| France (a) (1999) | SI | 78.1 | 4.3 | 72.8 | 21.9 | 12.2 | 9.7 | 1.1 |
| Germany (1998) | SI | 75.8 | 11.0 | 69.4 | 24.2 | 7.1 | 12.8 | 4.3 |
| UK (1999) | Tax | 83.3 | 73.5 | 9.8† | 16.7 | 3.4 | 11.2 | 2.1 |
| USA (1999) | Tax subsidised PI | 44.5 | 30.0 | 14.6 | 55.5 | 33.0 | 15.7 | 6.1 |

Data – Authors' research. Mossialos, 1999, European Observatory HiTs, OECD 2001. OECD 2002. Data should be interpreted with caution owing to the multiplicity of sources for this table.

*notes:*
(a) Drees 2001
† National Insurance

Table 1.6 shows a breakdown of UK healthcare expenditure in 1999 compared to France, Germany and the USA. In 2001, 73.5 per cent came from taxation, 9.8 per cent from national insurance contributions, 11.2 per cent from out-of-pocket spending, 3.4 per cent from private insurance and 2.1 per cent from other sources. If only the NHS revenues (UK) are considered, 80.4 per cent of income is from taxation, c. 12.1 per cent from NICs, four per cent from charges, three per cent from hospital interest receipts and one per cent from capital receipts.[19] In 1998-99, some 97 per cent of Scottish NHS expenditure came from general taxation and the NHS section of NICs. The remaining three per cent came from charges and other receipts.[20] It was estimated that 89 per cent of gross cost was met from taxation, c. nine per cent from NICs, two per cent from charges and other capital receipts.

*General taxation rates*[21]

The NHS in both England and Scotland is largely funded from the general tax pool, that is, direct and indirect taxes. Income tax is the major direct tax: it is charged at a starting rate of ten per cent, a basic rate of 22 per cent, and a higher rate of 40 per cent. The main source of indirect taxation is VAT—charged at 17.5 per cent. Expenditure on health amounted to 17 per cent of total government tax receipts in 1998.[22] The Scottish Parliament decides on Scottish spending priorities and is able to raise additional taxes, though it has not done so yet; tax rates are the same in Scotland and England.

*National (Social) Insurance*

National Insurance contributions (NICs), paid by employees and employers, are related to employee income and so are like a direct tax. A significant portion of the population incorrectly thinks existing national insurance contributions are largely spent on healthcare.[23] In fact only about ten per cent of healthcare funding[24] comes from national insurance; the remainder is from general taxation.[25] National Insurance is charged at ten per cent for employees (with a non-contributory allowance and maximum payment threshold) and 11.8 per cent for employers—soon to be raised to 11 per cent and 12.8 per cent respectively following Gordon Brown's latest budget, with the extra one per cent being strictly allocated to the NHS. In 2000-01, employers contributed 58 per cent while employees paid the balance. In 2000-2001, the mean average NIC per employee was £1,629. In the financial year 2001-2002 total income from NICs was £65,169 billion. Of this amount, roughly 80 per cent goes towards pension benefits.[26] By contrast, some 11.2 per cent (£7,304 billion) was 'allocated to' the NHS.[27]

According to some, the 'example of Scotland illustrates that higher levels of spending are achievable within the UK's tax (and NICs) funded system and at existing levels of taxation, by prioritising health over other areas of expenditure'.[28] Though plausible, we cannot agree with this statement, and refer readers back to Table 1.5, which sets out identifiable total managed expenditure in Scotland and the UK by programme for 2000-2001; in fact, health and personal social services account on Scotland for a slightly lower percentage of total managed expenditure than the UK.

*Private medical funding*

In comparison with other developed countries, private expenditure in both England and Scotland is low, though, as Tables 1.7 and 1.8 show, private expenditure as a percentage of total health expenditure has risen over the past two decades. Of EU member countries, only Luxembourg spends a lower level of GDP on private health care than the UK, and only Portugal and Luxembourg spend less per capita.[29] Although we do not have an accurate breakdown of total expenditure on health by funding source, it is reasonable to assume that the lower levels of private insurance (see below) in Scotland result in public sector sources being even more dominant north of the border than they are in England, perhaps even more so than in Portugal and Luxembourg.

### Table 1.7
#### Sources of healthcare funding in the UK as % of total expenditure on health, 1980-2000

| Funding source | 1980 | 1990 | 1995 | 1996 | 1997 | 1998 | 1999 |
|---|---|---|---|---|---|---|---|
| Public | 89.4 | 84.3 | 84.9 | 83.7 | 83.7 | 83.3 | 83.3 |
| Private | 10.6 | 15.7 | 15.1 | 16.3 | 16.3 | 16.7 | 16.7 |
| Out-of-pocket | 1.3 | 3.3 | 3.2 | 3.3 | 3.5 | 3.5 | 3.4 |
| VHI | 8.6 | 10.6 | 11.0 | 11.1 | 10.9 | 11.1 | 11.2 |

Source: Dixon and Robinson, 2002, p. 109; OECD Health Data 2002

### Table 1.8
#### Private expenditure trends, as % of total expenditure on health, 1980-99

| Countries | 1980 | 1990 | 1991 | 1992 | 1993 | 1994 | 1995 | 1996 | 1997 | 1998 | 1999 |
|---|---|---|---|---|---|---|---|---|---|---|---|
| France PS | 21.2 | 23.4 | 24.1 | 23.6 | 23.6 | 24.1 | 24.0 | 24.0 | 23.9 | 23.9 | 23.8 |
| OPPs | N/A | N/A | N/A | 11.7 | 11.5 | 11.2 | 11.1 | 10.6 | 10.5 | 10.3 | 10.1 |
| PI | N/A | N/A | N/A | 10.9 | 11.1 | 11.9 | 11.9 | 12.3 | 12.4 | 12.6 | 12.6 |
| Germany PS | 21.3 | 23.8 | 21.9 | 21.6 | 22.5 | 22.5 | 21.9 | 21.7 | 23.4 | 24.2 | N/A |
| OPPs | 10.3 | 11.1 | 10.8 | 10.7 | 11.4 | 11.4 | 10.9 | 11.0 | 12.2 | 12.8 | N/A |
| PI | 5.9 | 7.2 | 6.5 | 6.4 | 6.7 | 6.8 | 6.7 | 6.5 | 6.9 | 7.1 | N/A |

Notes:
PS: Private spending
OPPs: Out of pocket payments
PI: Private insurance
Figures for OPP and PI do not sum to the total private expenditure, as other sources of private expenditure are not shown.

*Insurance*

Private spending details are indicated in Table 1.7. In 1979 three million people in the UK had private insurance.[30] According to Laing's *Healthcare Market Review*, by 2001 this had risen to almost seven million people, with some 11.1 per cent of the population having supplementary private medical insurance (PMI).[31] PMI premiums are risk rated for individual policies and group rated for group policies. Income tax relief on private insurance premiums was abolished in the UK in 1997.

Access to private medical insurance is concentrated among the middle classes, and particularly in London and the South East of England where roughly 20 per cent are covered. Policies are mainly purchased by employers. The main insurers are BUPA (a provident society), PPP, Norwich Union and Standard Life Healthcare.[32] Additionally, around a third of a million people pay out of their pockets for private operations each year. Most NHS hospitals accept money from private patients to give them privileged access to the same beds, nurses, doctors and operating theatres; some NHS hospitals generate up to a quarter of their income from fee-paying patients.[33] The level of private sector healthcare activity (both insurance and provision) in Scotland is much smaller than in England; in 2001 only eight per cent of Scots had PMI or a 'non-insured medical expenses scheme', a figure lower than all other regions in Great Britain (average 12.3 per cent) excepting the North East where only six per cent were covered.[34] These figures suggest that poverty is a greater problem in the north.

*User charges*

Although 'free at the point of delivery', users in both England and Scotland are charged for prescriptions, as well as for dental and eye care. There are no charges for GP consultations or inpatient episodes, though patients can elect to pay out-of-pocket for certain amenities and privacy. Prescriptions are charged at a flat rate of £6.20 per item in both England and Scotland. However, approximately 85 per

cent of prescriptions are exempt from the charge.[35] In
Scotland 90 per cent of prescriptions were exempt from
payment in 2002. Not all of these were 'free', as regular
users may purchase pre-payment certificates. Charges are
payable for eye tests and for spectacles and contact lenses.
An eye test typically costs £15-£20, though there are a
number of exemptions from payment.[36] Dental patients in
both England and Scotland must pay 80 per cent of the cost
of dental care up to an annual maximum of £366.[37] There is
charge of £5.32 for a dental check up. Children and certain
benefits recipients receive free dental care. A number of
private pre-payment schemes exist in England and Scotland, designed to cover out-of-pocket charges for dental and
eye care, and other complementary treatment.[38]

### Healthcare Resource Distribution

Distribution of expenditure among forms of care (ambula-
tory care, hospital care, dentists, long-term nursing, drugs,
others) in the UK is as follows. Eighty-one per cent of total
NHS expenditure goes on hospital and community health
services (HCHS) and family health services (FHS) discretionary spending.[39] The remainder is divided between
capital spending (three per cent), family health services non
discretionary spending (including GP remuneration, dental
services ophthalmic services and charges for dispensing and
pharmaceutical services) (eight per cent), central health and
miscellaneous services (including public health functions
and departmental administration) (two per cent).[40] Tables
1.9 and 1.10 show that the division per capita between care
sectors is similar in England and Scotland; expenditure per
capita on FHS is slightly higher in Scotland, while expenditure on hospital services per capita is a little higher still.[41]

### Risk Adjustment

Risk adjustment is designed to promote geographical equity
in access (equal access for equal need) to healthcare services. In England, risk adjustment is commonly referred to
as 'weighted capitation', and is based on age, size of population, cost of delivering health care, and health need (split

into four needs sectors), relative to the national average.[42] The distinctive feature of Scotland is the major contrast between the urban Greater Glasgow health board, with all the problems associated with large conurbations, and the very remote Highland and Island boards, with markedly different problems of accessibility and dispersed population.[43] The Scottish risk adjustment mechanism[44] was replaced following the report 'Fair Shares for All' by Sir John Arbuthnott's Steering Group in 1999 to take account of these factors.

### Table 1.9
### UK, General Medical Services Expenditure per capita, and per household, 1975-2000/01

| Year | GMS Expenditure per capita (£ cash) | | At constant prices (index 1975/76=100) | |
|---|---|---|---|---|
| | England | Scotland | England | Scotland |
| 1975/76 | 6 | 7 | 100 | 100 |
| 1980/01 | 13 | 13 | 108 | 107 |
| 1990/01 | 41 | 40 | 182 | 168 |
| 1999/00 | 67 | 69 | 227 | 214 |
| 2000/01 | 69 | 72 | 229 | 225 |

Source: OHE, 2002, table 4.5
Notes: see OHE Compendium notes

### Table 1.10
### NHS Hospital gross expenditure (revenue and capital) per capita and household, UK, 1975/76 – 1999/00

| Year | Hospital expenditure per capita (£ cash) | | At constant prices (index 1975/76=100) | |
|---|---|---|---|---|
| | England | Scotland | England | Scotland |
| 1975/76 | 60 | 75 | 100 | 100 |
| 1999/00 | 450 | 573 | 153 | 156 |
| | Hospital expenditure per household (£ cash) | | At constant prices (index 1975/76=100) | |
| 1975/76 | 169 | 218 | 100 | 100 |
| 1999/00 | 1,080 | 1,318 | 130 | 125 |

Source: OHE, 2002, table 3.2.
Notes: see OHE Compendium notes

## Scottish and English Health Funding and Expenditure in an International Context

Based on the funding system and certain other health system characteristics such as the number of physicians and expenditure levels (see Tables 1.6, 4.1 and 4.2) Scotland, England and comparable countries can be divided into four groups (see Table 1.11).

### Table 1.11
### Income, expenditure and funding type

| Income and expenditure | High income Moderate expenditure | High income High expenditure | High income Very high expenditure |
|---|---|---|---|
| Countries and their funding mechanisms | Denmark (tax) UK (tax Scotland (tax) England (tax) | Canada (tax) Switzerland (SI) Netherlands (SI) France (SI) Germany (SI) | USA (PI, tax) |

*Source*: Hurst, 2000; also derived from World Bank Classifications (http://www.worldbank.org/data/countryclass/classgroups.htm)

*Notes*: PI = private insurance, SI = social insurance

The World Bank classifies all these countries as high income.[45] Following the example of Jeremy Hurst, Head of the OECD Health Policy Unit, we can divide them into three further groups.[46] The UK (England and Scotland) and Denmark, which have expenditure between US$ 1,200 and US$ 2,100 per capita, are in the first group of high-earning countries with low expenditure. Along with other OECD countries that fall into this group, they place an above-average (that average being about 75 per cent of total expenditure on health in 1998) reliance on public expenditure with taxation as the main source of funds.[47] Hospital ownership is mainly public and hospital doctors and GPs are paid mainly by salary or capitation (see Tables 4.1-4.6, pp. 44-50). Though health status in both countries is high and equity in access is officially according to need, there are significant waiting times for specialist care.[48] Healthcare expenditure relies heavily on politically controlled general taxation in England and Scotland—and there is an unwill-ingness to pay more tax.

The second group of high-earning countries includes Canada, France, Germany, the Netherlands and Switzer-land. Expenditure per capita is between US$1,500 and US $2,900. With other OECD countries that would fall into this group (Japan, Austria, Belgium, and Luxembourg) the share of public expenditure is also high (around the 1998 average of about 75 per cent) but, with the exception of Canada (decentralised tax), they are all based on compul-sory social health insurance. Among these countries, there are many different ways of organising healthcare funding through independent third-party payers (sickness funds), with various decision-making procedures and methods for the collection of contributions, risk pooling and redistribu-tion between funds. Meanwhile, healthcare provision is made by a mixture of public and private not-for-profit and profit-making organisations. Hospitals are more likely to be private and non-profit in this group and fee-for-service payment is more common. Health status is high and equity of access good. With the exception of Canada (2.1 per 1,000), the number of physicians per capita is at or above the OECD average (3.0 per 1,000) (see Tables 4.1-4.6 below).[49] Waiting times for specialists are shorter.[50] However, the Netherlands experiences significant waiting lists, and, compared to its neighbour, so does Canada. Rising health expenditure and supplier-induced demand are current concerns in these countries. Some consider the burden of social contributions on employers and employees in France, Germany and the Netherlands, too great.

The USA stands alone: with expenditure of over US$ 4,000 per capita, it is the highest spending country in the world. Voluntary employer-related private insurance is the main source of healthcare finance. This is supplemented by public schemes for children, the elderly and poor. Hospitals are mostly private non-profit. Managed care was introduced to improve cost control in the 1990s.[51]

## *Summary*

*On Funding*

- Scotland spends significantly more than England on healthcare
- Healthcare funding is predominantly public in both countries
- Taxation is the major source of healthcare funds in both countries
- Private (insurance) expenditure is significantly higher in England
- Expenditure per capita on family medical services is slightly higher in Scotland
- Hospital care expenditure per capita and per household is higher in Scotland.

# 2

# General Demographic/
# Environmental Indicators

## General Demographic and Environmental Health Inputs

Tables 2.1a and 2.1b show general health and demographic data for Scotland and England for the period 1976 to 2001. It is striking that trends in both countries have not consistently followed the same path. The population in England has been increasing (by c. six per cent since 1971) while that of Scotland has fallen by c. three per cent. The numbers of live births have fallen over the past 25 years in Scotland, but have risen in England, though English rates have in fact declined since 1991. Meanwhile Scottish birth rates have declined since 1981. Since 1995, the number of deaths has outweighed the number of births in Scotland, while the reverse is true in England and has been since at least 1981.

Age-standardised mortality has been falling steadily in both countries since 1976, but remains significantly higher in Scotland than in England. Both male and female life expectancy have risen steadily over the period, but again Scottish life expectancy remains significantly lower than that in England for both sexes; though it is perhaps worth noting that life expectancy in the USA (and Cuba, Costa Rica and the Czech Republic) is closer to that in Scotland than the rest of the UK.[1] Infant mortality reveals little difference between the two countries, both of which have cut rates significantly over the 25 years since 1976; since 1991 rates have been fractionally better in Scotland.

## Table 2.1a
## Key demographic and health indicators, England, 1976-2001
### (Numbers [thousands], rates)

| Year | Population | Live births | Deaths | Age standardised mortality | Male life expectancy at birth | Female life expectancy at birth | Infant mortality rates |
|------|-----------|-------------|--------|---------------------------|------------------------------|--------------------------------|------------------------|
| 1976 | 46,660 | 550.4 | 560.3 | 10,271 | N/A | N/A | 14.2 |
| 1981 | 46,821 | 598.2 | 541.0 | 9,298 | 71.1 | 77.0 | 10.9 |
| 1986 | 47,342 | 623.6 | 544.5 | 8,694 | 72.2 | 77.9 | 9.5 |
| 1991 | 48,208 | 660.8 | 534.0 | 7,941 | 73.4 | 79.0 | 7.3 |
| 1996 | 49,089 | 614.2 | 524.0 | 7,333 | 74.6 | 79.7 | 6.1 |
| 1997 | 49,284 | 608.2 | 519.1 | 7,190 | 74.9 | 79.9 | 5.9 |
| 1998 | 49,495 | 602.1 | 519.6 | 7,128 | 75.1 | 80.0 | 5.6 |
| 1999 | 49,753 | 589.5 | 519.6 | 7,062 | 75.4 | 80.2 | 5.7 |
| 2000 | 49,997 | 572.8 | 501.0 | 6,738 | N/A | N/A | 5.6 |
| 2001 | 49,181 | 563.7 | 496.1 | 6,665 | N/A | N/A | 5.4 (P) |
| 2002 | 49,342 | N/A | N/A | N/A | N/A | N/A | N/A |

*Source*: HSQ17 table 2.2
(P) provisional

25

## Table 2.1b
### Key demographic and health indicators, Scotland, 1976-2001
### (Numbers [thousands], rates)

| Year | Population | Live births | Deaths | Age-standardised mortality | Male life expectancy at birth | Female life expectancy at birth | Infant mortality rates |
|---|---|---|---|---|---|---|---|
| 1976 | 5,233 | 64.9 | 65.3 | 11,675 | 68.2 | 74.4 | 14.8 |
| 1981 | 5,180 | 69.1 | 63.8 | 10,849 | 69.1 | 75.3 | 11.3 |
| 1986 | 5,123 | 65.8 | 63.5 | 10,135 | 70.2 | 76.2 | 8.8 |
| 1991 | 5,107 | 67.0 | 61.0 | 9,254 | 71.4 | 77.1 | 7.1 |
| 1996 | 5,128 | 59.3 | 60.7 | 8,868 | 72.2 | 77.8 | 6.2 |
| 1997 | 5,123 | 59.4 | 59.5 | 8,623 | 72.4 | 77.9 | 5.3 |
| 1998 | 5,120 | 57.3 | 59.2 | 8,533 | 72.6 | 78.1 | 5.5 |
| 1999 | 5,119 | 55.1 | 60.3 | 8,618 | 72.8 | 78.2 | 5.0 |
| 2000 | 5,058 | 53.1 | 57.8 | 8,071 | N/A | N/A | 5.7 |
| 2001 | 5,064 | 52.5 | 57.4 | 7,930 | N/A | N/A | 5.5(P) |
| 2002 | 5,057 | N/A | N/A | N/A | N/A | N/A | N/A |

*Source:* HSQ17 table 2.2
(P) provisional

Age distribution is shown in Table 2.2. Scotland has a slightly different population pyramid, with fewer than England in the two lowest age-groups, roughly the same proportions in the 15-44 age-group, more in the 45-74 age-groups, and then fewer than England in the oldest group, presumably reflecting lower life expectancy.

### Table 2.2
### Population age-groups, 2001

| Age | England | Scotland |
|---|---|---|
| Total population | 49,181 | 5,064 |
| % 0-4 | 5.9 | 5.5 |
| % 5-15 | 14.2 | 13.7 |
| % 16-44 | 40.2 | 40.4 |
| % 45-64M / 59F | 21.3 | 21.8 |
| % 65M / 60F-74 | 10.8 | 11.5 |
| % 75 and over | 7.6 | 7.1 |

Source: HSQ 17, table 1.2

### Table 2.3
### Risk factors for morbidity and mortality in developed countries

| Risk Factor | Male ( %) | Female (%) |
|---|---|---|
| Smoking and oral tobacco | 17.1 | 6.2 |
| Alcohol | 14.0 | 3.3 |
| Blood Pressure | 11.2 | 10.6 |
| Cholesterol | 8.0 | 7.0 |
| Body Mass index | 6.9 | 8.1 |
| Low fruit and vegetable intake | 4.3 | 3.4 |

Source: Leon et al., 2002, taken from The World Health Report, 2002.

General environmental health inputs are important factors for morbidity and mortality and lead to ischaemic heart disease, stroke and cancer; our major killers (see Tables 2.3-2.4). For example, roughly one third of cancers are caused by smoking, and another third by diet.

Tables 2.5 and 2.6-2.8 show differences between England and Scotland in alcohol and tobacco consumption. Obesity rates, diet, cholesterol levels, rates of exercise, GDP, and income inequality are shown in Tables 2.9-2.15. While some data prove inconclusive (such as anthropometric profiles) it is clear from this information that health inputs are generally worse in Scotland than they are in England (although in England there is considerable regional variation from South to North). This has been recognised in Scotland as a major cause of concern.[2]

*Alcohol consumption*

Alcohol consumption is shown in Table 2.5. Low level alcohol consumption is in fact more prevalent in England than in Scotland, but the proportion consuming more than the recommended daily level of alcohol is much higher in Scotland than in England. In Scotland 46 per cent of men consume more than the recommended daily amount compared to 38 per cent in England. Thirty per cent of Scots women drink more than the recommended daily level compared to 22 per cent in England.

*Tobacco consumption*

Table 2.6 shows the prevalence of cigarette smoking in England and Scotland. Smoking is more prevalent in Scotland than in England, although this difference is more marked among women than among men. Scottish smokers often report heavier daily smoking.[3] In both countries there has been a decline in cigarette smoking, although this appears to have tailed off since the early 1990s. Among men there has been a 40 per cent decline in smoking in Scotland, compared to a 36 per cent decline in England. However, among women the decline has been slower in Scotland, 30 per cent compared to 34 per cent in England.

## Table 2.4
### Selected risk factors to health

| Risk Factor | Theoretical Minimum Exposure | Measured adverse outcomes of exposure |
|---|---|---|
| Blood Pressure | 115; SD 11mmHg | Stroke<br>IHD<br>hypertensive disease<br>other cardiac disease |
| Cholesterol | 3.8;SD 1 mmol/1 (147 SD 39 mg/d) | Stroke<br>IHD |
| Overweight | 21; SD 1 kg/m2 | Stroke<br>IHD<br>diabetes<br>osteoarhritis<br>endometrial cancer<br>postmenopausal breast cancer |
| Low fruit and vegetable intake | 600; SD 50 g intake per day for adults | Stroke<br>IHD<br>colorectal cancer<br>gastric cancer<br>lung cancer<br>oesophageal cancer |
| Physical inactivity | All taking at least 2.5 hours per week of moderate exercise or 1 hour per week of vigorous exercise | Stroke<br>IHD<br>colon cancer<br>breast cancer<br>diabetes |

Source: The World Health Report, 2002, p. 57.

## Table 2.5
### Alcohol consumption by sex and region, 2000, Great Britain

| MEN | Drank nothing last week | Maximum daily alcohol consumption (units) | | | Weighted base (000's) | Unweighted sample |
| --- | --- | --- | --- | --- | --- | --- |
| | | Up to four | Five to eight | More than eight | | |
| England | 25 | 37 | 17 | 21 | 17,604 | 5,707 |
| Scotland | 25 | 29 | 17 | 29 | 1,764 | 547 |
| Great Britain | 25 | 36 | 17 | 21 | 20,369 | 6,598 |

| WOMEN | Drank nothing last week | Up to three | Four to six | More than six | | |
| --- | --- | --- | --- | --- | --- | --- |
| England | 40 | 38 | 13 | 9 | 18,955 | 6,455 |
| Scotland | 41 | 29 | 18 | 12 | 2,026 | 664 |
| Great Britain | 40 | 37 | 13 | 10 | 22,054 | 7,499 |

*Source:* Office for National Statistics, *Living in Britain: Results from the General Household Survey 2000*, London: The Stationery Office: London, 2001.

*Notes:* Adults aged 16 and above. Alcohol consumption levels are based on the number of units of alcohol consumed on the heaviest drinking day during the previous week, the 'maximum daily amount'. Data are weighted for non-response. The weighted base is the base for percentages.

## Table 2.6
### Cigarette smoking, adults 16 and above, 1990-2000, England and Scotland compared

| | 1976 % | 1980 % | 1984 % | 1988 % | 1990 % | 1992 % | 1994 % | 1996 % | 1998 % | 2000 % |
|---|---|---|---|---|---|---|---|---|---|---|
| **MEN** | | | | | | | | | | |
| England | 45 | 42 | 35 | 32 | 31 | 29 | 28 | 28 | 28 | 29 |
| Scotland | 50 | 46 | 43 | 36 | 33 | 34 | 31 | 33 | 33 | 30 |
| Great Britain | 46 | 42 | 36 | 33 | 31 | 29 | 28 | 29 | 28 | 29 |
| **WOMEN** | | | | | | | | | | |
| England | 37 | 36 | 32 | 30 | 28 | 27 | 25 | 27 | 26 | 25 |
| Scotland | 43 | 42 | 35 | 37 | 35 | 34 | 29 | 31 | 29 | 30 |
| Great Britain | 38 | 37 | 32 | 30 | 29 | 28 | 26 | 28 | 26 | 25 |

*Source: Coronary Heart Disease Statistics, British Heart Foundation, 2003, p. 80.*

*Table 2.7: Cigarette smoking among children aged 11-15, by sex, 1982 – 1998, England and Scotland*

| | | 1982 % | 1984 % | 1986 % | 1988 % | 1990 % | 1992 % | 1993 % | 1994 % | 1996 % | 1998 % |
|---|---|---|---|---|---|---|---|---|---|---|---|
| MALES | **England** | | | | | | | | | | |
| | Regular smoker | 11 | 13 | 7 | 7 | 9 | 9 | 8 | 10 | 11 | 9 |
| | Occasional smoker | 7 | 9 | 5 | 5 | 6 | 6 | 7 | 9 | 8 | 8 |
| | Used to smoke | 11 | 11 | 10 | 8 | 7 | 6 | 6 | 7 | 7 | 9 |
| | Tried smoking | 26 | 24 | 23 | 23 | 22 | 22 | 22 | 21 | 22 | 20 |
| | Never smoked | 45 | 44 | 55 | 58 | 56 | 57 | 57 | 53 | 53 | 54 |
| | **Scotland** | | | | | | | | | | |
| | Regular smoker | 15 | 16 | 10 | | 11 | 10 | | 11 | 14 | 11 |
| | Occasional smoker | 8 | 8 | 4 | | 8 | 6 | | 8 | 8 | 8 |
| | Used to smoke | 13 | 14 | 11 | | 9 | 9 | | 9 | 9 | 9 |
| | Tried smoking | 27 | 24 | 25 | | 23 | 24 | | 23 | 24 | 24 |
| | Never smoked | 37 | 39 | 50 | | 49 | 52 | | 50 | 45 | 48 |
| FEMALES | **England** | | | | | | | | | | |
| | Regular smoker | 11 | 13 | 12 | 9 | 11 | 10 | 11 | 13 | 15 | 12 |
| | Occasional smoker | 9 | 9 | 5 | 5 | 6 | 7 | 9 | 10 | 10 | 8 |
| | Used to smoke | 10 | 10 | 10 | 9 | 7 | 7 | 10 | 8 | 9 | 10 |
| | Tried smoking | 22 | 22 | 19 | 19 | 18 | 19 | 18 | 17 | 18 | 18 |
| | Never smoked | 49 | 46 | 53 | 59 | 58 | 57 | 53 | 52 | 48 | 51 |
| | **Scotland** | | | | | | | | | | |
| | Regular smoker | 14 | 17 | 14 | | 12 | 13 | | 13 | 14 | 13 |
| | Occasional smoker | 10 | 9 | 6 | | 8 | 8 | | 10 | 9 | 11 |
| | Used to smoke | 13 | 12 | 12 | | 11 | 13 | | 11 | 13 | 14 |
| | Tried smoking | 21 | 22 | 22 | | 20 | 20 | | 22 | 20 | 22 |
| | Never smoked | 41 | 40 | 45 | | 49 | 45 | | 44 | 44 | 40 |

*Source: Coronary Heart Disease Statistics*, British Heart Foundation, 2003, p. 78.

Smoking among children is also higher for Scotland than England (Table 2.7). It appears to have declined in both countries in boys, but among girls in both countries there appears to have been a slight increase throughout the 1990s. Albeit starting from a lower level, this increase has been more pronounced in England than Scotland.

Though smoking patterns are a cause for real concern, overall smoking among adults in the UK is lower than the EU average (see Table 2.8).

### Table 2.8
### Percentage regular daily smokers, adults 15 years and above, 1992-2000, UK compared to EU average

|            | 1992 | 1994 | 1996 | 1998 | 2000 |
|------------|------|------|------|------|------|
|            | %    | %    | %    | %    | %    |
| UK         | 28   | 27   | 28   | 27   | 27   |
| EU Average | 30   | 29   | 29   | 29   | 29   |

Source: British Heart Foundation Coronary Heart Disease Statistics, 2003

## Diet

Table 2.9 shows the consumption of key food groups in England and Scotland. In spite of Scotland's reputation for being the country of two fish-and-chip suppers a day, the differences in total fat and saturated fat consumption are not significant. There is also very little difference in the consumption of salt. The only difference appears to be in the consumption of fruit and vegetables, which is lower for Scotland. There is considerable regional variation in England, with people in the South East consuming 193g of fruit and 170g of vegetables per day. This is 35 per cent more fruit and 31 per cent more vegetables consumed in the South East of England relative to Scotland, compared to 23 per cent more fruit and 25 per cent more vegetables consumed in England as a whole relative to Scotland. However, data from the National Diet and Nutrition Survey suggest that the percentage eating the recommended five portions of fruit and vegetables per day is the same for Scotland as for London and the South East of England, and higher than for the rest of England and Wales.[4] David Leon et al. note that the Scottish Health Survey 1998 shows that children in Scotland were more likely to have eaten fruit every day than English children (57 per cent versus 50 per cent). They caution that there may be an especially important knock-on effect of low fruit and vegetable consumption, because it is likely to increase the negative effects of exposure to other risk factors such as smoking.[5]

*Table 2.9*
**Household consumption of (a) energy, fat, saturated fat, (b) fruit and vegetables, and (c) salt, England and Scotland compared, 2000**

|  |  | Scotland | England |
|---|---|---|---|
| **(a) Energy and Fat** |  |  |  |
| | *Consumption per day* |  |  |
| Energy | (kcal) | 1,650.0 | 1,760.0 |
| | (MJ) | 6.9 | 7.4 |
| *Percentage of food energy from fats* |  |  |  |
| Total fat | | 38.6 | 38.0 |
| Saturated fatty acids | | 15.7 | 14.9 |
| **(b) Fruit and Vegetables** |  |  |  |
| | *Consumption per person per day* |  |  |
| Fruit (grams) | | 132.0 | 159.0 |
| Vegetables – excluding potatoes (grams) | | 125.0 | 158.0 |
| **(c) Salt** |  |  |  |
| | *Consumption per person per day* |  |  |
| Sodium | (grams) | 2.6 | 2.6 |
| Salt | (grams) | 6.5 | 6.6 |

Source: Tables B5 and B11, Department for Environment, *Food and Rural Affairs National Food Survey 2000*, London: The Stationery Office, 2001.

Conversion factor: salt (g) = sodium (g) x 2.52

## Body Weight and Obesity

Table 2.10 shows body weight patterns in England and Scotland as measured by the 1998 Health Surveys. The data (not shown) reveal that there are no marked differences in mean body mass index[6] for any age/sex group. However, they also show that Scotland has a lower prevalence of overweight men (42.6 per cent) compared to England (45.3 per cent) but a higher prevalence of obese men (19.6 per cent) compared to England (17.4 per cent). Among

women of all age-groups, there appears to be little difference in overweight or obesity between England and Scotland. The only group in which any significant difference was
revealed was Scottish women aged 16-24, who showed
greater prevalence of overweight and obesity (30.6 per cent
were found to be overweight or obese compared to 27.3 per
cent in England). The picture presented for waist/hip ratio[7]
(WHR), the measure of central obesity, is a little more
complex (Table 2.11). Among men the prevalence of a raised
WHR is slightly less likely in Scotland than in England.
Among women this is reversed—women in Scotland are
more likely to have a raised WHR than women in England.

Among children there appears to be no significant
recorded difference in body weight or obesity between
England and Scotland (data not shown).

### Table 2.10
### Adult body mass index in Scotland and England, 1998

| BMI | Body Mass Index (kg/m²) | | | | | |
|---|---|---|---|---|---|---|
| | <20 | 20-25 | 25-30 | 30-40 | >40 | Obese (over 30) |
| | % | % | % | % | % | % |
| MEN | | | | | | |
| Scotland | 4.5 | 33.3 | 42.6 | 18.7 | 0.8 | 19.6 |
| England | 3.6 | 33.6 | 45.3 | 16.7 | 0.7 | 17.4 |
| WOMEN | | | | | | |
| Scotland | 6.4 | 39.4 | 32.1 | 20.1 | 2.0 | 22.1 |
| England | 6.5 | 40.6 | 31.6 | 19.3 | 2.0 | 21.3 |

*Source*: The Scottish Health Survey, 1998.

### Table 2.11
### Adult waist/hip ratio in Scotland and England, 1998

| | Waist/Hip Ratio % | |
|---|---|---|
| | Men | Women |
| | WHR 0.95 and above | WHR 0.85 and above |
| Scotland | 24.4 | 20.0 |
| England | 26.5 | 17.6 |

*Source*: The Scottish Health Survey, 1998.

*Physical Activity*

Table 2.12 shows that between the ages of 16 and 54 men in
Scotland are as physically active as men in England, but
that over the age of 55 men in England are likely to be more
active. This pattern is mirrored in the female populations,
with women in England aged between 55 and 74 more likely
to be active than women of the same age cohort in Scotland,
although for younger women there was no difference. As
cardiovascular diseases are age-related, this may well be
significant.

**Table 2.12**
**Summary of overall participation in physical activities
in Scotland and England**

| | 16-24 | 25-34 | 35-44 | 45-54 | 55-64 | 65-74 | All ages |
|---|---|---|---|---|---|---|---|
| | Percentage active at recommended weekly level[8] | | | | | | |
| | % | % | % | % | % | % | % |
| MEN | | | | | | | |
| Scotland | 55 | 48 | 40 | 33 | 26 | 14 | 38 |
| England | 58 | 48 | 43 | 36 | 32 | 17 | 40 |
| WOMEN | | | | | | | |
| Scotland | 33 | 31 | 34 | 29 | 19 | 8 | 27 |
| England | 32 | 31 | 32 | 30 | 21 | 12 | 27 |

*Source:* Scottish Health Survey 1998.

*Raised Cholesterol*

David Leon *et al.* note that the 1998 Health Surveys for
England and Scotland suggested that mean total cholesterol
was similar in Scotland and England for both sexes at all
ages. This overall picture hides certain detail. Scottish men
in the 35-64 age-group have a slightly higher proportion of
those with a cholesterol level of 6.5mmol/L or greater. But
the proportion is lower for Scots men than English, in the
65-74 age-group. HDL cholesterol levels were the same for
those sampled in both countries.[9]

*Raised Blood Pressure*

Leon *et al.* also note that hypertension is lower for both
males and females in Scotland than England.[10] Scottish
prevalence rates are 33.1 per cent for men and 28.4 per cent

for women. Meanwhile English rates are 40.1 per cent for men and 29.4 per cent for women. Higher English preva- lence rates apply for all age-groups with the exception of the 45-64 group. Mean systolic blood pressure was also slightly lower in Scotland than in England over all ages and both sexes.[11] The 'mean diastolic blood pressure was also lower in Scotland than in England for both males (73.5mm Hg compared to 76.0mm Hg) and females (69.5mm Hg com- pared to 71.7mm Hg).'[12]

*GDP per head*[13]

There is a well-established link between income and health; increasing income is linked with better health.[14] Table 2.13 shows GDP per head at current basic prices. Scotland has had a lower per capita GDP than England for the past decade. As might be expected, GDP per capita has increased throughout the UK. The levels of increase are broadly similar for England and Scotland: England's GDP has risen 64 per cent and Scotland's has risen 66 per cent compared to a UK average of 65 per cent. GDP per head rose in Scotland throughout the early 1990s, until by 1995 it was higher than GDP per head in both England and the UK. Since 1995 it has fallen, and in 1999 stood in almost the same relation to England and the UK as it had done in 1989.

*Income inequality*[15]

Average income in Britain has risen since the 1970s but income inequality has widened dramatically, and after stab- ilising in the early 1990s has increased since 1997.[16] There have been few studies on the differences in level of income- related inequality, but those there are indicate that income inequality is greater in England than in Scotland. They indicate that income inequality has increased in Scotland, in line with Britain overall, but remains slightly lower. Table 2.14 shows the Gini Coefficient for disposable income for Scotland compared to Great Britain as a whole.[17]  An- alysis of Department of Work and Pensions (DWP) figures

## Table 2.13
### Gross Domestic Product (GDP) at current basic prices (as at 23/10/02)

| | 1989 | 1990 | 1991 | 1992 | 1993 | 1994 | 1995 | 1996 | 1997 | 1998 | 1999 |
|---|---|---|---|---|---|---|---|---|---|---|---|
| **GDP per head (£)** | | | | | | | | | | | |
| UK | 8,053 | 8,712 | 9,050 | 9,404 | 9,852 | 10,372 | 10,842 | 11,462 | 12,118 | 12,750 | 13,213 |
| England | 8,069 | 8,692 | 9,020 | 9,384 | 9,852 | 10,349 | 10,771 | 11,384 | 12,141 | 12,845 | 13,278 |
| Scotland | 7,544 | 8,321 | 8,814 | 9,217 | 9,614 | 10,168 | 10,818 | 11,162 | 11,429 | 12,117 | 12,512 |
| **GDP per head:** | | | | | | | | | | | |
| **Indices (UK less Extra-Regio = 100)** | | | | | | | | | | | |
| UK | 100 | 100 | 100 | 100 | 100 | 100 | 100 | 100 | 100 | 100 | 100 |
| England | 102.3 | 101.8 | 101.6 | 101.6 | 101.9 | 101.8 | 101.4 | 101.8 | 102.3 | 102.4 | 102.4 |
| Scotland | 95.6 | 97.5 | 99.3 | 99.8 | 99.4 | 100.0 | 101.9 | 99.8 | 96.3 | 96.6 | 96.5 |

- Estimates of regional GDP in this table are on a residence basis, where income of commuters is allocated to where they live, rather than their place of work
- Provisional
- Components may not sum to totals as a result of rounding
- The GDP for Extra-Regio comprises compensation of employees and gross operating surplus which cannot be assigned to regions

*Source: Regional Trends 37*, Office for National Statistics, 2002.

by the New Policy Institute for the same period suggest that the disparity between the tenth income percentile and the 90th income percentile, i.e. the richest and poorest sections of the community, grew by eight per cent in Scotland, while it remained fairly stable for England and Wales.[18] However, it still remains lower than the level of inequality in England and Wales.[19] A recent study comparing income-related health inequalities seems to suggest that this difference obtains for Scotland and England compared directly, although the data are not comprehensive[20] (Table 2.15). This study also plotted income inequality against self-reported health in the countries of Great Britain and found greater income-related health inequality in Scotland and Wales compared to England, in spite of lower income inequality. This suggested to the authors that what income inequality there was in Scotland and Wales had a greater proportional impact on health inequality than in England. This echoes findings on a European scale, which have shown that Britain has wider health inequalities than would be expected for its level of income inequality compared to countries such as Sweden.[21]

### Table 2.14
### Gini Coefficient for disposable income†
### Scotland and GB compared, 1994/5 – 1999/2000

|  | Gini Coefficient (%) disposable income | | | | | |
|  | 1994-95 | 1995-96 | 1996-97 | 1997-98 | 1998-99 | 1999-00 |
|---|---|---|---|---|---|---|
| Scotland | 31 | 30 | 30 | 31 | 31 | 33 |
| Great Britain | 33 | 33 | 33 | 34 | 35 | 34 |

† There are a number of income measures for which the Gini Coefficient can be calculated, largely depending on whether the incomes have been adjusted for tax and benefits. Disposable income is used here as it is the only level for which data for Scotland are available.

Source: Scottish Economic Statistics, 2002.

**Table 2.15**
***Gini Coefficient England and Scotland***

|  | Gini (Income 0.72) | | |
|  | 1993 | 1994 | 1995 |
| --- | --- | --- | --- |
| Scotland | 0.281 | 0.278 | 0.281 |
| England | 0.285 | 0.287 | 0.285 |

*Source*: Gravelle and Sutton, 2003.

## Summary

### On Population and Environmental Inputs

- Alcohol consumption is higher in Scotland than that in England
- Tobacco consumption is higher in Scotland
- Diet (measured by fruit, vegetable and fat consumption) in Scotland is poorer than that in England
- There is little difference in overweight or obesity between England and Scotland. The only group in which any significant difference was revealed was Scottish women aged 16-24, who showed greater prevalence of overweight and obesity
- Rates of exercise in Scotland are often lower than those in England (aged group dependent)
- Blood cholesterol levels are higher in England
- Hypertension is more prevalent in England
- Systolic and diastolic blood pressure is lower in Scotland over all ages and both sexes
- Income inequality is less pronounced in Scotland
- But there is greater income-related health inequality in Scotland

# 3

# Healthcare Benefits Package

All legal residents in England and Scotland are entitled to receive care from the NHS. The National Health Service Act 1977 charges the Secretary of State with a general responsibility to provide services 'to such an extent as he considers necessary to meet all reasonable requirements'.[1] But unlike an insurance policy, there is no clear contract laying down the services that people's tax and national insurance payments entitle them to receive. The British National Formulary indicates which drugs are available for sale in the UK. It is not a positive list, but does indicate which drugs are not available on prescription from the NHS.[2] Unlike the English, and following one of the most famous post-devolution decisions by the Scottish Parliament, Scots are entitled to personal and nursing care paid for by the government, though this does not cover housing and living costs.[3]

## Equity and Equality

Equity in both access to and the funding of health care has been examined by academics working on the ECuity project.[4] Findings indicate that access to GP and specialist care is equitable in the UK, but that NHS funding is perhaps not.[5] Taken together, direct and indirect taxes are mildly progressive—that is, they weigh more heavily on the better off. However, if the distribution of the tax burden is considered by quintile, it is clear that regressive indirect taxes account for a higher proportion of taxation for some. The result is that the lowest quintile pays 40 per cent of income on taxation, while the upper quintile pays 36 per cent.[6]

The introduction of explicit rationing through NICE has gone some way to spelling out entitlements to treatments.

40

NICE was set up as a Special Health Authority for England and Wales on 1 April 1999. It is an independent organisation, responsible for providing national guidance on treatments and care for those using the NHS in England and Wales.[7] All 302 primary care trusts and 274 NHS Trusts in England must make decisions about which treatments to fund. Different trusts make different decisions. This means that whether or not you receive the treatment that you need is determined by where you live. By providing national guidance NICE aims to eliminate such inequities. However, despite the fact that since 1 January 2002 the NHS has had a statutory obligation to provide funding for NICE-approved technologies once a doctor has recommended it to his or her patient, NICE rulings do not amount to concrete benefits; there is still significant geographical variation in treatment.[8] Until its replacement in January 2003 by NHS Quality Improvement Scotland, the Scottish equivalent to NICE was the Health and Technology Board for Scotland (HTBS), founded in April 2000 to supplement the Scottish Intercollegiate Guidelines Network (SIGN), which has been running since 1993. The HTBS advises the NHS in Scotland on the clinical and cost-effectiveness of innovations in health care including new drugs and treatments. None of the clinical guidance boards have supplementary powers, nor can their recommendations affect funding. SIGN, for example, has produced over forty sets of guidelines since its inception. However, as for NICE, these guidelines are not accompanied by any implementation powers or resources, and there is some doubt as to their level of implementation.[9] HTBS had also been plagued by debates as to its efficacy, in part for the reasons mentioned above, but also as it has been dismissed as an evaluation body for the work of its English counterpart.[10]

Civitas research, using Prescription Cost Analysis data from the Department of Health website, suggests that implementation of NICE guidance is patchy. NICE and the HTBS have not succeeded in ironing out the postcode lottery for treatment with drugs and new technologies. Here is part of the text of a letter to the *BMJ* by Edinburgh-based experts David Cameron (a medical oncologist) and Michael Dixon (a consultant breast surgeon):

EDITOR: We had understood that one of the intentions of the National Institute for Clinical Excellence (NICE) was to rationalise the introduction of new drugs and technologies across the United Kingdom so that NHS patients would have equitable access. This has plainly not happened. We illustrate the problem with three recently licensed drugs, imatinib, irinotecan, and trastuzumab.

Imatinib has yet to be appraised by the National Institute for Clinical Excellence, but our local haematologists completed the paperwork for approval by Lothian Health Board's drug evaluation panel. The drug was not approved. Shortly afterwards the Scottish Medicines Consortium issued guidance to indicate that it should be made available: we await the result of an appeal to the drug evaluation panel. Meanwhile patients in Fife can get it.

Irinotecan was approved by the National Institute for Clinical Excellence and the Health Technology Board for Scotland. However, the drug evaluation panel for Lothian has rejected it despite knowing the decisions of the institute and the board on the grounds that the improved survival does not justify the cost. If the patients live in the west of Scotland, however, they can receive it. In Aberdeen doctors are allowed to prescribe it but without any additional funding, so that expenditure on irinotecan competes with that on other drugs.

Trastuzumab was approved by the institute after a year's deliberation, and then by the Health Technology Board for Scotland. It is already available in the west of Scotland; but recognising that the real decision about its availability in the east of Scotland lies with the Lothian Health Board, we have to carry out a detailed assessment of the total cost before applying to the drug evaluation panel. The only reason we have any optimism about its decision is that some funding may already have been identified.

The current system seems no more equitable than previously...[11]

# 4

# Health System Resources and Organisation of NHS in Scotland and England

Since its establishment on 5 July 1948, the NHS has aimed to provide a comprehensive range of health services to UK citizens, free at the point of use and paid for from taxation. Devolution resulted in the creation of the Scottish Parliament, which took full powers in July 1999 with Donald Dewar as First Minister. Health care, along with education, housing and a number of other policy areas, is a devolved matter.[1] The ultimate responsibility for providing health services lies with the Secretary of State for Health in England (John Reid, MP) and the Scottish Minister for Health and Community Care (Malcolm Chisholm). Ministers are supported by their respective ministries—the Department of Health in England and the Scottish Executive Department of Health in Scotland.[2] The following section sets out some evidence on health system resources and organisation in Scotland and England. Data for other countries are included to aid comparison.

Forms of hospital ownership, methods of payment and the number of physicians per capita, are shown in Table 4.1. Most importantly for our purposes, Scotland and England present a similar picture of public ownership of hospitals, similar payment methods (though not for hospital care),[3] and an absence of the money-follows-the-individual patient principle.[4]

## Table 4.1
### Hospital ownership and healthcare resource allocation characteristics

| Country Characteristic | France | Germany | UK | England | Scotland | USA |
|---|---|---|---|---|---|---|
| **Hospital Ownership** | Public and private | Public and private | Public | Public | public | Private mostly non-profit |
| **Public private split (%)** | Public - 65<br>Private - 20<br>Non-profit - 15 | Public - 55<br>Private - 7<br>Non-profit - 38 | Public - 94<br>Private - 6 | Public - >94<br>Private - <6 | Public - <94 +<br>Private - >6 | Public - 24<br>Private - 15<br>Non-profit - 61 |
| **GP payment** | FFS + some extra billing | FFS | Capitation + expenses | Capitation + expenses[5] | Capitation + expenses | Mixed<br>Managed care<br>Some FFS |
| **Money follows individual patient (accountability)** | Yes | Yes | Not yet | Not yet<br>Very limited effective choice[6] | No | Yes<br>Managed care |
| **Hospital payment** | Prospective global budgets + activity related £ | DRGs<br>Dual financing | Activity related purchaser provider contracts | Activity related purchaser provider contracts | Public<br>Integrated model | Mixed |

*Source:* Civitas research. European Observatory HIT reports, and Mossialos and Le Grand, 1999. US figures from American Hospital Association.

## Table 4.2
### Other system features

| Country Characteristic | France | Germany | UK | Scotland | England | USA |
|---|---|---|---|---|---|---|
| Equity in access (a) | Good | Good | Good | Good | Good | 15% Uninsured (c. 40 million) |
| GP Gatekeeping | No | Very weak | Yes | Yes | Yes | HMO |
| National Concerns | High expenditure | High expenditure | Waiting lists Queue hopping by privately insured | Waiting lists Public Health | Waiting lists Public Health | High expenditure Uninsured Managed care restrictions |

*Source:* Civitas research
(a) *Source:* Wagstaff, *et al.*, 1993 and Civitas commissioned author's reports, 2002.
Note that equity in access does not imply that patients receive high quality and appropriate care.

The existence of GP gatekeeping as well as specific national concerns—including waiting lists, high expenditure, informal payments, managed care restrictions and uninsured individuals—are presented in Table 4.2. NHS patients in both Scotland and England are obliged to see a GP in order to obtain a referral before seeing a specialist. Most GP referrals are made to the local hospital, following contractual relationships between the hospital and health authority/health board or PCT/LHCC.[7] Waiting times are a major concern to patients and therefore politicians in both Scotland and England. Table 4.3 shows data on in-patient or day-case admission waiting lists and times taken from the latest edition of *Social Trends*. The most striking difference between the countries shown is the performance of Wales.

*Table 4.3*
*Waiting times in the UK compared, March 2002*

| Country | Less than 6 months (% total) | 6-12 months (% total) | 12 months or longer (% total) | Total Waiting (thousands) |
|---|---|---|---|---|
| England | 77 | 21 | 2 | 1,022 |
| Wales | 63 | 23 | 14 | 71 |
| Scotland | 81 | 17 | 3 | 72 |

Notes: 'Waiting times refer to people waiting for admission on either an in-patient or a day-case basis and the length of time they had waited to date. At 31 March... There are differences between countries in the ways that waiting times are calculated.'

Source: *Social Trends 33*, 2003 edn, pp. 152-53.

As waiting times vary widely by procedure and also by trust, comparison of headline rates in England and Scotland should be treated with caution.[8] The total number of patients waiting for admission in England (end of third quarter 2002) was 1,048,100 (c. one in 47 of the population).[9] Of these almost 237,000 waited for six months or longer for ordinary or day-case admissions. The number of English patients waiting over one year at the end of September 2002 was 16,700.[10] In Scotland, at the end of 2001, 81,968 (c. one in 61 of the population) were on a waiting list. The median length of wait for first outpatient appointment has increased in Scotland from 41 days in 1995 to 55 days in 2002,[11] while the median wait in England is c. 51 days.[12]

Across English trusts, an average of 76 per cent of patients see a specialist within 13 weeks from the date they were given their appointment. The corresponding figure in Scotland is only 72 per cent.[13] The median wait for inpatient appointments in Scotland was 33 days in the year ending March 2002.[14] In March 2003, the *Sunday Times* found that the percentage of people who have their hospital inpatient appointment (all specialties) within six months of the decision to admit is 79 per cent in England and 92 per cent in Scotland. [15]

NHSScotland and the NHS in England are the largest employers in both countries, but examination of human resources reveals differences between them. Roughly 132,000 people work for NHSScotland, including over 63,000 nurses, midwives and health visitors and over 8,500 hospital doctors.[16] Just under one million people work for the NHS in the England. In whole-time equivalents, NHS England employs over 782,000, including 99,000 hospital medical staff, 388,000 nurses and midwives.[17] Both countries are in the midst of drives to significantly increase numbers of nurses, specialists and GPs.[18] Table 4.6 shows that there are more physicians per 1,000 population in Scotland than in England. Both the number of GPs and of specialists per 1,000 population is higher in Scotland. The average GP patient list size is also much lower in Scotland. England has slightly more advanced medical technology equipment than Scotland, though both countries have significantly lower provision than many other OECD countries. Tables 4.4 and 4.5 indicate the number of physicians, specialists, GPs, nurses, hospital beds, and the availability of CT and MRI scanners in comparable countries.

The number of NHS acute hospital beds per 1,000 population is lower in England's 377 NHS Trust hospitals than that provided in the 28 Scottish hospitals. In 2001-2002, there were 108,000 beds of all types in England (c. 2.2 per 1,000), while in Scotland there were 17,693 (c. 3.53 per 1,000). The same pattern applies for nurses too; in 2001, there were 5.4 WTE qualified nurses in England and 7.3 in Scotland.

## Table 4.4
### Healthcare resources

| Country Characteristic | France | Germany | UK | Scotland | England | USA |
|---|---|---|---|---|---|---|
| Practising physicians per 1,000 pop (a) | 3.00 | 3.60 | 1.80 | N/A | N/A | 2.80 |
| International comparison | Average | High | Low | Low | Low | Low |
| Specialists per 1,000 pop | 1.50 | 2.40 | 1.60 | 1.50 | 1.20 | 1.40 |
| GPs per 1,000 pop | 1.50 | 1.00 | 0.60 | 0.69 | 0.55 | 0.80 |
| Nurses per 1,000 pop | 6.00 (97) | 9.30 | 5.30 | | 5.20 | 8.30 |
| Acute beds 1,000 pop | 4.20 | 6.40 | 3.30 | 3.53 | 2.20 | 3.00 |

*Source*: Civitas research. OECD Health Data 2002.

*Notes*: Data definitions for the Scotland and England columns are not wholly comparable with the remaining columns, with the result that UK rates are sometimes higher than those in Scotland.

(a) Source OECD 2002. Variations in definitions between indicators and between countries mean that 'practising physicians' is not simply a combination of GPs and specialists. See OECD 2002 'Sources and Methods', Health Employment.

## Table 4.5
### Healthcare technology resources

| Country Characteristic | Denmark | England | France | Germany | Netherlands | Switzerland | Scotland | UK | USA |
|---|---|---|---|---|---|---|---|---|---|
| CT Scanners per million | 10.90 | 5.66 | 9.60 | 17.10 | 7.20 (92) | 18.50 | 5.60 | 3.60 | 13.60 |
| MRIs per million | 6.6 (00) | 3.49 | 2.50 (97) | 6.20 (97) | 3.90 | 13.00 | 3.13 | 3.90 (99) | 8.10 |
| Radiation treatment Equipment per million | N/A | 3.80 | 7.60 (97) | 4.70 (96) | N/A | 5.00 (98) | 3.00 | 3.50 (98) | 3.80 (92) |
| Public investment in medical facilities as % total expenditure on health (THE) | 2.80 | N/A | 2.40 | 2.60 | N/A | 2.70 | N/A | 2.50 | 0.40 |
| per capita purchasing power parity (PPP) | 68 | N/A | 50 | 63 | N/A | 76 | N/A | 39 | 15 |

Source: Civitas research. NHSScotland Cancer Scenarios (p. 307); OECD Health Data 2002. National Cancer Services Analysis Team, NHS Executive (North West) website (www.cancernw.org.uk/) accessed 18 March 2003.

(a) Beds in nursing homes are not included. Source OECD 2002.

## Table 4.6
### Total number of medical staff, unrestricted GP principals and average list sizes, nurses, and acute beds (1998/9)

| Country | England | | Scotland | |
|---|---|---|---|---|
| All NHS doctors (2001) | 99,169 | | 11,953 | |
| Hospital medical staff numbers (2001) | 67,840 | | 8,573 | |
| Hospital medical staff WTE (2001) | 59,920 | | 7,665 | |
| Hospital medical staff WTE per 1000 pop | 1.2 | | 1.5 | |
| GPs numbers (1999) (unrestricted GP principals) WTE | 25,900 | | 3,536 | |
| Patient list (98) | 1,867 | | 1,449 | |
| GPs per 1,000 pop | 0.52 | | 0.71 | |
| Total nurses, midwives, etc (2001) | 493,730 | | 52,203 | |
| Qualified nurses total WTE (2001) | 266,170 | | 36,425 | |
| Qualified nurses per 1,000 pop | 5.4 | | 7.3 | |
| Acute beds (DoH form KH03) | 108,535 | (2001) | 17,693 | (2002) |
| Acute beds 1,000 pop | 2.2 | | 3.53 | |
| Acute beds occupation rates | 84.5% | | 81.3% | |
| Mean stay in acute hospital (days) | 6 | | 7.2 | |
| Median length of wait for first outpatient appointment (days) | 51 | | 55 | |

*Source*: Department of Health HES 2001-2002 Table 21. Main operations; HPSSS Tables D5 and D6; OHE compendium of statistics; DoH, Hospital......1991-2001, DoH, 2002; ISD NHSiS resource - online Annual Trends Workforce and Activity. ISD Annual trends in Activity, waiting Times and Waiting Lists; Directorate of Access & Choice Access Delivery (Waiting Times Analysis) Team, 21 March 2003.

*Notes*: rates per thousand are determined by using the following populations: England (49,400,000); Scotland (5,010,000).

## *Further Resources/Supply Data*

Tables 4.7 to 4.16 present further Scottish and English hospital services data taken from the Office of Health Economics' (OHE) Compendium of Health Statistics 2002.[19] Tables 4.17 to 4.19 present further family health services (GP) data, again from the OHE 2002 Compendium.

## *Hospital Services*

### Table 4.7: Medical and dental staff employed in NHS hospitals, UK, 1970-2000

| Year | Number of medical and dental staff | | Staff per 100,000 population | |
|---|---|---|---|---|
| | England + Wales | Scotland | England + Wales | Scotland |
| 1970 | 23,299 | 3,224 | 48 | 54 |
| 1980 | 34,298 | 5,163 | 69 | 99 |
| 1990 | 44,041 | 5,940 | 87 | 116 |
| 1995 | 52,324 | 6,642 | 101 | 129 |
| 1996 | 54,257 | 6,974 | 104 | 136 |
| 1997 | 57,257 | 7,295 | 110 | 142 |
| 1998 | 59,294 | 7,364 | 113 | 144 |
| 1999 | 61,081 | 7,535 | 116 | 147 |
| 2000 | 63,050 | 7,578 | 119 | 148 |

*Source*: Yeun, OHE, 2002, table 3.4

### Table 4.8: NHS Available hospital beds and FCEs per medical and dental staff, 1970-2000/01

| Year | Available beds per staff | | Finished consultant episodes (FCEs) per staff | |
|---|---|---|---|---|
| | England + Wales | Scotland | England + Wales | Scotland |
| 1970 | 20 | 20 | 229 | 217 |
| 1980 | 11 | 11 | 176 | 150 |
| 1990/91 (a) | 6 | 9 | 213 | 154 |
| 1995/96 | 4 | 6 | 226 | 146 |
| 1996/97 | 4 | 6 | 221 | 138 |
| 1997/98 | 4 | 5 | 213 | 134 |
| 1998/99 | 3 | 5 | 214 | 132 |
| 1999/00 | 3 | 4 | 211 | 128 |
| 2000/01 | 3 | 4 | 206 | 126 |

Source: Yeun, OHE, 2002, table 3.5

### Table 4.9: NHS hospitals' nurses and midwifery staff, (WTE) UK, 1970-2000

| Year | Nurses and midwifery staff ('000s) | | Staff per 100,000 population | |
|------|------------------|----------|-------------------|----------|
|      | England + Wales | Scotland | England + Wales | Scotland |
| 1990 | 380.8 | 56.2 | 749 | 1,102 |
| 1995 | 355.2 | 46.2 | 685 | 900 |
| 1996 | 356.1 | 45.7 | 685 | 892 |
| 1997 | 354.0 | 45.2 | 678 | 882 |
| 1998 | 355.9 | 44.7 | 679 | 872 |
| 1999 | 362.6 | 44.7 | 688 | 874 |
| 2000 | 370.5 | 44.4 | 700 | 869 |

*Source*: Yeun, OHE, 2002, table 3.6

### Table 4.10: NHS available hospital beds and FCEs per nursing and midwifery staff, 1980-2000/01

| Year | Available beds per staff | | FCEs per staff | |
|------|------------------|----------|-------------------|----------|
|      | England + Wales | Scotland | England + Wales | Scotland |
| 1980 | 1.0 | 1.1 | 15.3 | 14.5 |
| 1990/91 | 0.6 | 0.9 | 21.8 | 16.2 |
| 1995/95 | 0.6 | 0.9 | 33.3 | 21.1 |
| 1999/00 | 0.6 | 0.7 | 35.6 | 21.6 |
| 2000/01 | 0.5 | 0.7 | 35.1 | 21.5 |

*Source*: Yeun, OHE, 2002, table 3.7

### Table 4.11: Number of hospital medical staff in Scotland and England

| Year | Number of hospital medical staff | | Number per 100,000 | |
|------|---------|----------|---------|----------|
|      | England | Scotland | England | Scotland |
| 1991 | 49,895 | 6,706 | 103 | 131 |
| 1995 | 55,348 | 7,339 | 113 | 143 |
| 1999 | 63,548 | 8,154 | 128 | 159 |
| 2000 | 65,374 | 8,226 | 131 | 161 |
| 2001 | 67,838 | 8,573 | 135 | 168 |

*Source*: Yeun, OHE, 2002, table 3.8

## Table 4.12: Average daily available and occupied beds in NHS hospitals, UK 1980-2000/01

| Year | Average daily available beds per 1,000 population | | Average daily occupied beds '000s | | Bed occupancy rate | |
|------|---------|----------|---------|----------|---------|----------|
|      | England | Scotland | England | Scotland | England | Scotland |
| 1980 | 7.7 | 11.2 | 307 | 48 | 80 | 84 |
| 1990/01 | 5.4 | 9.9 | 229 | 41 | 83 | 82 |
| 1999/00 | 3.8 | 6.5 | 154 | 28 | 83 | 84 |
| 2000/01 | 3.8 | 6.3 | 156 | 27 | 84 | 83 |

*Source*: Yeun, OHE, 2002, tables 3.12 and 3.15

## Table 4.13: FCEs/discharges and deaths, UK, 1980-2000/01

| Year | FCEs/discharges and deaths '000s | | FCEs/discharges and deaths per bed | |
|------|---------|----------|---------|----------|
|      | England | Scotland | England | Scotland |
| 1980 | 6,036 | 774 | 15.8 | 13.4 |
| 1990/01 | 8,782 | 912 | 34.4 | 18.0 |
| 1999/00 | 12,197 | 965 | 65.5 | 28.8 |
| 2000/01 | 12,265 | 957 | 65.9 | 29.8 |

*Source*: Yeun, OHE, 2002, table 3.16

## Table 4.14: Average inpatient length of stay in NHS hospitals, all specialties, UK, 1980-2000/01

| Year | Average inpatient length of stay in days | | Index (1951=100) | |
|------|---------|----------|---------|----------|
|      | England | Scotland | England | Scotland |
| 1951 | 46.0 | 43.0 | 100 | 100 |
| 1980 | 19.0 | 23.0 | 41 | 53 |
| 1990/01 | 10.0 | 17.0 | 22 | 40 |
| 1999/00 | 5.0 | 7.5 | 11 | 17 |
| 2000/01 | 5.1 | 7.4 | 11 | 17 |

*Source*: Yeun, OHE, 2002, table 3.19

*Table 4.15*
**Hospital outpatient clinics: total attendances, UK, 1980-2000/01**

| Year | Outpatient total attendances '000s | | Per 1,000 | |
|---|---|---|---|---|
| | England | Scotland | England | Scotland |
| 1980 | 50,994 | 5,321 | 1,028 | 1,024 |
| 1990/01 | 55,775 | 5,925 | 1,096 | 1,168 |
| 1999/00 | 62,476 | 6,424 | 1,186 | 1,255 |
| 2000/01 | 62,663 | 6,451 | 1,184 | 1,261 |

*Source*: Yeun, OHE, 2002, table 3.39

*Table 4.16:*
**Hospital outpatient clinics: new cases, UK, 1980-2000/01**

| Year | New outpatient cases '000s | | Per 1,000 | |
|---|---|---|---|---|
| | England | Scotland | England | Scotland |
| 1980 | 18,146 | 1,999 | 366 | 385 |
| 1990/01 | 20,950 | 2,381 | 412 | 471 |
| 1999/00 | 26,866 | 2,734 | 510 | 534 |
| 2000/01 | 26,972 | 2,766 | 509 | 541 |

*Source*: Yeun, OHE, 2002, table 3.40

## Family Health Services

*Table 4.17*
**UK, number of unrestricted principals 1980-2001**

| Year | Number of unrestricted principals | | Per 100,000 population | |
|---|---|---|---|---|
| | England + Wales | Scotland | England + Wales | Scotland |
| 1980 | 23,184 | 2,959 | 46.7 | 57.0 |
| 1990 | 27,257 | 3,359 | 53.7 | 65.9 |
| 1995 | 28,421 | 3,524 | 54.8 | 68.6 |
| 2000 | 29,479 | 3,707 | 55.7 | 72.5 |
| 2001 | 29,628 | 3,755 | 55.7 | 73.5 |

*Source*: Yeun, OHE, 2002, table 4.8

### Table 4.18
### Number and list size of unrestricted principals UK, 1991-2001

| Year | Number of unrestricted GPs | | Average list size per unrestricted GP | |
|------|---------|----------|---------|----------|
|      | England | Scotland | England | Scotland |
| 1991 | 25,686  | 3,380    | 1,938   | 1,580    |
| 1995 | 26,702  | 3,524    | 1,887   | 1,506    |
| 1999 | 26,710  | 3,697    | 1,846   | 1,441    |
| 2000 | 27,704  | 3,707    | 1,853   | 1,425    |
| 2001 | 27,843  | 3,755    | 1,841   | 1,409    |

*Source*: Yeun, OHE, 2002, table 4.10

### Table 4.19
### UK, people aged 65 and over and those aged 75 and over, by unrestricted principal, UK 1991-2001

| Year | Number of over 65s per unrestricted GP | | Number of over 75s per unrestricted GP | |
|------|---------|----------|---------|----------|
|      | England | Scotland | England | Scotland |
| 1991 | 297     | 226      | 133     | 97       |
| 1995 | 290     | 221      | 129     | 93       |
| 1998 | 289     | 214      | 135     | 94       |
| 1999 | 291     | 212      | 138     | 93       |
| 2000 | 282     | 212      | 134     | 94       |

*Source*: Yeun, OHE, 2002, table 4.12

## Summary

### On Resources

- Healthcare resources are predominantly publicly owned and managed in both countries
- There is more private provision in England
- The NHS is the largest employer in both England and Scotland
- There are fewer doctors, dentists, nurses, and midwives per capita in England than Scotland

- There are more GPs per capita in Scotland (lists sizes are smaller in Scotland)
- The number of elderly (those over 65 and those over 75) on GP lists is lower on average in Scotland
- Hospital care expenditure per capita and per household is higher in Scotland
- Expenditure per capita on FMS is slightly higher in Scotland
- There are more consultant cardiologists per head in Scotland
- There are slightly more specialist and medical oncologists per head in Scotland
- There are fewer acute beds per capita in England than Scotland
- There are fewer available beds per medical, dental, and nursing staff in England
- There are fewer radiotherapy/diagnostic (MRI/CT/LinAc) machines per capita in Scotland
- The number of specialist stroke units per million is significantly lower in England
- There is significant geographical variation in resource provision in both countries

*On Activity*

- There are more finished consultant episodes per medical and dental staff in England
- FCEs/discharges and deaths per bed are significantly higher in England
- Bed occupancy rates are similar, though higher in England
- Average length of stay is longer in Scotland
- Total attendances (per 1,000) at hospital outpatient clinics are higher in Scotland.

# 5

# Healthcare Outcomes in
# England and Scotland

- Cause Specific Mortality
- Coronary Heart Disease (CHD) Outcomes [1]
- Stroke Outcomes
- Cancer Outcomes

*Snapshot of mortality rates*

It is generally accepted that mortality is a poor measure of
the performance of a healthcare system, largely because so
much mortality can be explained by the non-medical factors
discussed in section 2 above, which lie beyond the scope of
the health system (see inputs in model in Figure 1 of the
introduction).[2] Nevertheless, we include the following
tables, 5.0.1A-B (cause specific mortality rates [per 100,000]
and rankings of 6/17 Western European countries),[3] as they
clearly show the poor position of both England and Scotland
in an international perspective. It is also clear that mortality for the Scots is worse than for the English for both sexes
and for causes for which Leon *et al.* collected data (see
tables 5.0.2A-D). The position of Scottish women is as bad,
if not worse, than that for Scottish men. In comparison with
other Western European countries, in general terms
mortality in Scotland has 'far more in common with other
parts of the UK than with any other specific countries'.
More positively, Leon *et al.* note that the picture for certain
external factors (including suicide and road traffic accidents) is better in Scotland and England than many other
Western European countries.[4]

## Table 5.0.1A
### Number of deaths and age-standardised mortality rates, per 100,000, by main cause, sex and country, UK, 1999

| MALES Cause | Number of deaths | | Age-standardised mortality rates (a) | |
|---|---|---|---|---|
| | England and Wales | Scotland | England and Wales | Scotland |
| All causes | 264,229 | 28,605 | 878 | 1,069 |
| Infectious and parasitic diseases | 1,850 | 237 | 7 | 9 |
| All cancers | 69,543 | 7,474 | 232 | 275 |
| Stomach Cancer | 3,821 | 368 | 13 | 13 |
| Colorectal Cancer | 7,496 | 883 | 25 | 33 |
| Lung Cancer | 18,342 | 2,305 | 61 | 84 |
| Prostate Cancer | 8,533 | 769 | 27 | 28 |
| Diabetes Mellitus | 2,815 | 317 | 9 | 12 |
| Circulatory system | 105,120 | 11,606 | 43 | 429 |
| Hypertensive disease | 1,490 | 169 | 5 | 6 |
| Coronary heart disease | 63,317 | 7,122 | 208 | 263 |
| Cerebrovascular disease | 20,711 | 2,494 | 67 | 92 |
| Respiratory system | 43,776 | 3,804 | 141 | 142 |
| Pneumonia | 23,391 | 1,782 | 76 | 68 |
| BEA (b) | 2,731 | 221 | 9 | 8 |
| Digestive system | 9,808 | 1,386 | 34 | 53 |
| Ulcer of stomach and duodenum | 1,955 | 170 | 6 | 6 |
| Chronic liver disease + cirrhosis | 2,904 | 564 | 11 | 22 |
| External causes of injury + poisoning | 10,466 | 1,507 | 38 | 59 |
| Motor vehicle traffic accidents | 2,126 | 226 | 8 | 9 |
| Suicide and self-inflicted harm | 2,840 | 500 | 11 | 19 |

Source: OHE Compendium of Health Statistics 2002 (source based on WHO Mortality Database)
Notes: (a) per 100,000. (b) Bronchitis, chronic and unspecified, emphysema and asthma.

## Table 5.0.1B

| FEMALES Cause | Number of deaths | | Age-standardised mortality rates | |
|---|---|---|---|---|
| | England and Wales | Scotland | England and Wales | Scotland |
| All causes | 291,819 | 31,676 | 586 | 707 |
| Infectious and parasitic diseases | 1,771 | 261 | 4 | 6 |
| All cancers | 64,592 | 7,315 | 162 | 190 |
| *Stomach cancer* | 2,318 | 282 | 5 | 7 |
| *Colorectal Cancer* | 7,111 | 815 | 16 | 19 |
| *Lung Cancer* | 11,151 | 1,656 | 29 | 44 |
| *Breast cancer* | 11,604 | 1,129 | 32 | 32 |
| Diabetes Mellitus | 3,148 | 353 | 6 | 8 |
| Circulatory system | 114,14 | 13,181 | 209 | 269 |
| *Hypertensive disease* | 1,834 | 184 | 3 | 4 |
| *Coronary heart disease* | 51,803 | 6,215 | 97 | 131 |
| *Cerebrovascular disease* | 35,342 | 4,291 | 62 | 84 |
| Respiratory system | 54,000 | 5,066 | 95 | 103 |
| *Pneumonia* | 35,897 | 2,744 | 58 | 51 |
| *BEA (b)* | 2,085 | 220 | 5 | 6 |
| Digestive system | 11,903 | 1,401 | 25 | 34 |
| *Ulcer of stomach and duodenum* | 2,056 | 167 | 4 | 4 |
| *Chronic liver disease + cirrhosis* | 1,814 | 332 | 6 | 12 |
| External causes of injury + poisoning | 6,073 | 943 | 16 | 25 |
| *Motor vehicle traffic accidents* | 816 | 90 | 3 | 3 |
| *Suicide and self-inflicted harm* | 850 | 137 | 3 | 5 |

*Source:* OHE Compendium of Health Statistics 2002 (source based on WHO Mortality Database)
*Notes:* (a) per 100,000. (b) Bronchitis, chronic and unspecified, emphysema and asthma

60

## Table 5.0.2A
### Cancer mortality rates (per 100,000) and rankings of 6/17 Western European countries for men aged 15-74, 1991-1995

| Rank | Oesophageal cancer | | Stomach cancer | | Colo-rectal cancer | | Pancreatic cancer | | Lung cancer | |
|---|---|---|---|---|---|---|---|---|---|---|
| | Country | Rate | County | Rate | Country | Rate | Country | Rate | Country | Rate |
| 1 | Scot (1) | 24 | Scot (6) | 21 | Den (3) | 38 | Den (4) | 16 | Scot (1) | 126 |
| 2 | Fr (2) | 20 | Ger (11) | 16 | Scot (5) | 36 | Scot (6) | 16 | Den (5) | 101 |
| 3 | E+W (5) | 14 | E+W (12) | 14 | Ger (7) | 27 | Swit (8) | 14 | Fr (10) | 48 |
| 4 | Den (6) | 13 | Swit (14) | 12 | E+W (8) | 26 | Ger (12) | 13 | Swit (11) | 77 |
| 5 | Swit (7) | 12 | Den (16) | 11 | Swit (9) | 26 | Fr (13) | 12 | E+W (12) | 75 |
| 6 | Ger (13) | 9 | Fr (17) | 11 | Fr (13) | 22 | E+W (16) | 11 | Ger (14) | 70 |

*Source:* Leon, *et al.*, 2002, Appendix II.

*Notes*: figures in parentheses are rankings out of 17 Western countries (Austria, Belgium, Denmark, Finland, France, Germany, Ireland, Italy, Netherlands, Norway, Portugal, Spain, Sweden, Switzerland, UK – England and Wales, UK – Northern Ireland, UK – Scotland). Standardised to EASR.

## Table 5.0.2B
### Other causes mortality rates (per 100,000) and rankings of 6/17 Western European countries for men aged 15-74, 1991-1995

| Rank | IHD | | Cerebrovascular D | | Ch, Obst Pul disorder | | Liver Cirrhosis | | All causes | |
|---|---|---|---|---|---|---|---|---|---|---|
| | Country | Rate | County | Rate | Country | Rate | Country | Rate | Country | Rate |
| 1 | Scot (1) | 311 | Scot (3) | 59 | Den (3) | 43 | Ger (3) | 39 | Scot (1) | 854 |
| 2 | E+W (5) | 213 | Ger (7) | 44 | Scot (4) | 37 | Den (6) | 30 | Den (4) | 773 |
| 3 | Den (7) | 190 | Den (8) | 43 | E+W (6) | 32 | Fr (7) | 29 | Ger (6) | 758 |
| 4 | Ger (10) | 154 | E+W (10) | 41 | Ger (7) | 28 | Swit (10) | 19 | E+W (10) | 683 |
| 5 | Swit (12) | 117 | Fr (16) | 29 | Swit (12) | 23 | Scot (11) | 19 | Fr (11) | 682 |
| 6 | Fr (17) | 63 | Swit (17) | 25 | Fr (17) | 14 | E+W (14) | 10 | Swit (16) | 600 |

Source: Leon et al., 2002, Appendix II.

## Table 5.0.2C
### Cancer mortality rates (per 100,000) and rankings of 6/17 Western European countries for women aged 15-74, 1991-1995

| Rank | Oesophageal cancer | | Stomach cancer | | Colo-rectal cancer | | Pancreatic cancer | | Lung cancer | | Breast cancer | |
|---|---|---|---|---|---|---|---|---|---|---|---|---|
| | Country | Rate | County | Rate | Country | Rate | Country | Rate | Country | Rate | Country | Rate |
| 1 | Scot (1) | 11 | Scot (5) | 9 | Den (1) | 28 | Den (5) | 13 | Scot (1) | 66 | Den (1) | 55 |
| 2 | E+W (4) | 5 | Ger (6) | 9 | Scot (5) | 23 | Scot (7) | 11 | Den (2) | 60 | Scot (4) | 48 |
| 3 | Den (5) | 5 | Den (11) | 7 | Ger (7) | 18 | Swit (9) | 11 | E+W (5) | 36 | E+W (7) | 44 |
| 4 | Swit (9) | 3 | E+W (14) | 6 | E+W (10) | 17 | Ger (12) | 8 | Swit (9) | 19 | Swit (8) | 41 |
| 5 | Fr (13) | 2 | Swit (16) | 5 | Swit (12) | 15 | E+W (13) | 7 | Ger (13) | 14 | Ger (10) | 36 |
| 6 | Ger (14) | 2 | Fr (17) | 4 | Fr (17) | 12 | Fr (16) | 6 | Fr (15) | 10 | Fr (13) | 33 |

*Source:* Leon, *et al.*, 2002, Appendix II.

*Table 5.0.2D*

**Other causes mortality rates (per 100,000) and rankings of 6/17**
**Western European countries for women aged 15-74, 1991-1995**

| Rank | IHD | | Cerebrovascular D | | Ch, Obst Pul disorder | | Liver Cirrhosis | | All Causes | |
|---|---|---|---|---|---|---|---|---|---|---|
| | Country | Rate | County | Rate | Country | Rate | Country | Rate | Country | Rate |
| 1 | Scot (1) | 128 | Scot (2) | 51 | Den (1) | 39 | Ger (2) | 16 | Scot (1) | 498 |
| 2 | E+W (5) | 77 | Den (6) | 32 | Scot (4) | 27 | Den (4) | 14 | Den (2) | 473 |
| 3 | Den (6) | 74 | E+W (7) | 31 | E+W (5) | 19 | Fr (6) | 13 | E+W (5) | 398 |
| 4 | Ger (10) | 51 | Ger (9) | 27 | Ger (10) | 9 | Scot (7) | 12 | Ger (7) | 348 |
| 5 | Swit (13) | 33 | Fr (16) | 15 | Swit (11) | 8 | Swit (12) | 8 | Swit (15) | 283 |
| 6 | Fr (17) | 15 | Swit (17) | 14 | Fr (16) | 5 | E+W (13) | 6 | Fr (16) | 275 |

*Source*: Leon *et al.*, 2002, Appendix II.

*Notes*: figures in parentheses are rankings out of 17 Western countries. Standardised to EASR.

In light of the 2002-2006 Scottish Budget which called for a 'step-change in life expectancy for Scots', in comparison to other developed countries, Leon *et al.* briefly discuss 'Step-change' in mortality; defining it as a change in the ranking of a country[5] by five places, for all causes of mortality at working age, between the periods 1955-60 and 1990-1995. Scotland has not achieved a 'step-change', but England (along with Denmark, Norway and the Netherlands) has seen a 'step-change' deterioration for women in relation to the other countries studied. Ireland and Denmark have also experienced 'step-change' deterioration for men.[6]

It is perhaps best to think of the healthcare sector as having a 'repairing' role.[7] We have attempted to identify those changes in health status strictly attributable to the activities of the healthcare system.[8] In some cases death can be avoided or significantly delayed if appropriate medical treatment is given in time. In such instances, mortality can be used as a healthcare system performance indicator. We collated available measures of medical performance for the two main killers—cancer and diseases of the circulatory system, including coronary heart disease and stroke. For cancer we compared post-diagnosis one-year and five-year survival rates, which offer a good indication of the performance of a healthcare system in relation to cancer care.

The frequency of use of medical interventions of recognised effectiveness can also be employed as an indicator of healthcare system performance. For example, two types of heart disease operations, coronary artery bypass grafting (CABG) and percutaneous transluminal coronary angioplasty (PTCA), are considered effective treatments in relieving pain, preventing heart attacks and prolonging life.[9] PTCA has seen increases in prevalence in recent years but, according to a study by the ageing related disease (ARD) team at the OECD, there is considerable variation between OECD countries.[10] We collected CABG and PTCA rates for Scotland and England.

## 5.1 CHD Outcomes and Treatment

Cardiovascular disease statistics we aimed to gather:

- Coronary heart disease, incidence and mortality
- Number of specialist units (revascularisation facilities)
- Revascularisation rates
- Number of coronary artery bypass grafts (CABGs per million population (pmp))
- Number of percutaneous transluminal coronary angioplasty (PTCA) pmp
- The extent of blood cholesterol concentration monitoring
- Blood pressure (or 'hypertension') monitoring
- Action taken on blood pressure (e.g. for angina—if systolic pressure > 160 mm Hg, or systolic pressure > 140 mm Hg and cholesterol > 5.5 mmol/1[11]
- Tobacco consumption status
- Management of obesity (diet therapy use)

*Heart Disease in England and Scotland—Overview*

The UK has historically suffered higher incidence and mortality from coronary heart disease compared to the rest of Western Europe, and within the UK Scotland has suffered, and continues to suffer, from more instances of coronary heart disease than England. Services for the treatment of heart disease are generally acknowledged to have been haphazardly delivered and unevenly provisioned in both countries.[12] In recent years there has been greater recognition by both governments of CHD as a major health problem and of the inadequacy of service delivery compared to similar countries. The recognition of CHD as a major health priority has manifested itself in different responses across the devolved governments. A National Service Framework (NSF) for coronary heart disease was introduced in March 2000 and has been rolled out across England. The NSF sets out standards, appropriate interventions, service models and targets for all aspects of CHD from population-based prevention to acute care and rehabilitation. It has been argued that the introduction of the NSF in England has already led to significant improvements in care; an overall increase in the number of coronary revascularisations, reductions in waiting times and improved rates of thrombolysis have all been directly attributed to its implementation.[13] The NSF has not been implemented in any of the devolved countries. In Scotland a strategy for coronary heart disease was published in October 2002. This covers many of the issues addressed in the NSF, such as clinical audit, information technology systems and staffing. It is too early to assess the impact of this strategy in Scotland.

*Mortality*

Scotland has a higher mortality rate for coronary heart disease, when compared to England (see Tables 5.1.1A - 5.1.2 below). Although Scottish mortality has been declining steadily over the past 20 years, at approximately the same rate as that in England, it remains significantly higher— currently standing at 261 per 100,000 for men and 98 per 100,000 for women. This compares to an English mortality rate of 207 per 100,000 for men and 70 per 100,000 for women. The UK averages are 213 and 68 per 100,000 for men and women respectively. When compared to those for France and Germany, the mortality rates for Scotland are significantly higher than Germany, although mortality rates in England are closer to those in Germany. Both are considerably higher than those in France. Scotland has the second highest rate of mortality from CHD in Western Europe[14] and the UK as a whole has the third highest rate of mortality—only Ireland and Finland have higher rates. However, Leon and his team found that, for men and women of working age, Scotland has the highest rates. Furthermore, in spite of the decline in mortality from CHD in England and Scotland, rates of decline since the mid-seventies have also been slower than for many other developed countries. Finland, for example, enjoyed a 44 per cent decline in mortality in men aged 35-74 between 1988 and 1998, Denmark a 49 per cent fall and Australia a 46 per cent fall. Scotland's death rate for the same period fell 38 per cent and England's fell 39 per cent. The same figure in the female population was 43 per cent in Finland, 46 per cent in Denmark, and 52 per cent in Australia compared to 39 per cent in Scotland and 41 per cent in England.[15]

*Incidence*
Incidence is the number of first-ever cases reported in a year, while prevalence is the proportion of a population at a particular time who have ever reported symptoms of a particular condition, and measures the extent of a particular disease in a country. Comparable data on health disease incidence and prevalence are notoriously difficult to gather,[16] and incidence rate is especially problematic.[17] While no conclusive data on prevalence or incidence of all forms of CHD in England and Scotland exists, health surveys, national data and local studies all provide information on various aspects of morbidity that can be used to give an indication of trends in incidence and prevalence (see Table 5.1.3). Comparison of these sources would seem to suggest that there is generally higher incidence of CHD in Scotland than in England, particularly when compared to Southern England, but also in relation to Northern England.

Data from the Health Survey for England and the Scottish Health Survey[18] for comparable ages also suggest a greater prevalence of coronary heart disease in Scotland (Table 5.1.4).

## Table 5.1.1A
### Age-standardised death rates per 100,000 population, 1990-2000, men

| Men 35-45 | 1990 | 1991 | 1992 | 1993 | 1994 | 1995 | 1996 | 1997 | 1998 | 1999 | 2000 | 2001 |
|---|---|---|---|---|---|---|---|---|---|---|---|---|
| UK | 393 | 379 | 364 | 357 | 325 | N/A | 292 | 295 | 260 | 244 | 226 | 213 |
| England | 377 | 363 | 349 | 338 | 307 | 297 | 281 | 260 | 251 | 234 | 218 | 207 |
| Scotland | 481 | 468 | 458 | 453 | 408 | N/A | 371 | 347 | 332 | 318 | 289 | 261 |

## Table 5.1.1B
### Age-standardised death rates from CHD per 100,000 population, 1990-2001, women

| Women 35-74 | 1990 | 1991 | 1992 | 1993 | 1994 | 1995 | 1996 | 1997 | 1998 | 1999 | 2000 | 2001 |
|---|---|---|---|---|---|---|---|---|---|---|---|---|
| UK | 145 | 141 | 134 | 131 | 120 | N/A | 104 | 98 | 93 | 85 | 78 | 68 |
| England | 137 | 133 | 127 | 119 | 109 | 104 | 99 | 92 | 89 | 82 | 73 | 70 |
| Scotland | 201 | 195 | 182 | 180 | 160 | N/A | 140 | 136 | 129 | 118 | 109 | 98 |

## Table 5.1.2
### Age-standardised death rates per 100,000 population from CHD, selected countries compared, 1998

|  | Men 35-74 | Women 35-74 |
|---|---|---|
| UK | 260 | 93 |
| England | 251 | 89 |
| Scotland | 302 | 129 |
| Germany | 200 | 69 |
| France | 83 | 21 |

*Source*: British Heart Foundation Statistics Database 2003

## Table 5.1.3
### Incidence of myocardial infarction (MI), adults aged between 30 and 69, latest available year, UK studies compared

| Source | Study | Year | Place | Sex | Age-group | Incidence/ 100,000 | Mortality/ 100,000 |
|---|---|---|---|---|---|---|---|
| Volmink et al., 1998 | OXMIS | 1994/1995 | Oxfordshire | Men | 30-69 | 292 | 120 |
| | | | | Women | 30-69 | 94 | 44 |
| Tunstall-Pedoe et al., 1999 | MONICA | 1985/94 | Glasgow | Men | 35-64 | 777 | 365 |
| | | | | Women | 35-64 | 265 | 123 |
| Tunstall-Pedoe et al., 1999 | MONICA | 1983/93 | Belfast | Men | 35-64 | 695 | 279 |
| | | | | Women | 35-64 | 188 | 79 |
| Lampe et al., 2000 | BRHS | 1983/95 | Great Britain | Men | 45-59a | 950 | 426 |

Table compiled by British Heart Foundation

Original Sources: Volmink, J.A., Newton, J.N., Hicks, N.R., Sleight, P., Fowler, G.H. and Neil, H.A.W., on behalf of the Oxford Myocardial Infarction Incidence Study Group (1998) Coronary event and case fatality rates in an English population: results of the Oxford myocardial infarction incidence study. Heart 80; 40-44; Tunstall-Pedoe, H., Kuulasmaa, K., Mahonen, M., Tolonen, H., Ruokokoski, E. and Amouyel, P., for the WHO MONICA Project (1999). Contribution of trends in survival and coronary-event rates to changes in coronary heart disease mortality: 10 year results from 37 WHO MONICA Project populations. Lancet 353; 1547-1557; Lampe, F.C., Whincup, P.H., Wannamathee, S.G., Shaper, A.G., Walker, M. and Ebrahim, S., (2000). The natural history of prevalent ischemic heart disease in middle-aged men. European Heart Journal 21; 1052-1062.

Notes: (a) at start of follow up (1983/85). Some rates were age-standardised. See original sources for methods of age-standardisation and definitions of MI.

### Table 5.1.4
### Prevalence of CHD,*
### by age and sex, England and Scotland, 1998

|               | Age |       |       |
|---------------|-----|-------|-------|
| Reported      | 45-54 | 55-64 | 65-74 |
| CHD           | %   | %     | %     |
| **Men**       |     |       |       |
| Scotland      | 6.6 | 16.1  | 27.3  |
| England       | 4.3 | 13.6  | 20.2  |
| **Women**     |     |       |       |
| Scotland      | 4.1 | 11.9  | 20.9  |
| England       | 1.8 | 6.3   | 12.5  |

*Source*: Scottish Health Survey 1998, Health Survey for England—Cardiovascular Disease 1998

* Reported as ever having heart attack or angina as diagnosed by a doctor

## CHD Risk Factors

Smoking increases CHD risk. It has been estimated that 20 per cent of male CHD deaths and 17 per cent of deaths in women are caused by smoking. Tables 5.1.5 and 5.1.6 show smoking rates in Scotland and England (see population and environmental inputs section above for brief comparison between England and Scotland of these and other risk factor data).

### Table 5.1.5
### Cigarette smoking, adults 16 and above, 1990-2000,
### England and Scotland compared

|               | 1990 | 1992 | 1994 | 1996 | 1998 | 2000 |
|---------------|------|------|------|------|------|------|
|               | %    | %    | %    | %    | %    | %    |
| **Men**       |      |      |      |      |      |      |
| England       | 31   | 29   | 28   | 28   | 28   | 29   |
| Scotland      | 33   | 34   | 31   | 33   | 33   | 30   |
| Great Britain | 31   | 29   | 28   | 29   | 28   | 29   |
| **Women**     |      |      |      |      |      |      |
| England       | 28   | 27   | 25   | 27   | 26   | 24   |
| Scotland      | 35   | 34   | 29   | 31   | 29   | 30   |
| Great Britain | 29   | 28   | 26   | 28   | 26   | 25   |

### Table 5.1.6
### Percentage regular daily smokers, adults 15 years and above, 1992-2000, UK compared to EU average

|            | 1992 | 1994 | 1996 | 1998 | 2000 |
|------------|------|------|------|------|------|
|            | %    | %    | %    | %    | %    |
| UK         | 28   | 27   | 28   | 27   | 37   |
| EU Average | 30   | 29   | 29   | 29   | 29   |

*Source*: British Heart Foundation Coronary Heart Disease Statistics, 2003

It has been estimated that up to 30 per cent of deaths from CHD are owing to unhealthy diets.[19] More serious still, about 36 per cent of CHD deaths in men and 38 per cent in women are due to low levels of physical activity.[20] High consumption of alcohol also increases CHD risk.[21] About 14 per cent of CHD deaths in men and 12 per cent in women are caused by raised blood pressure. Blood cholesterol levels are directly related to CHD risk; about 45 per cent of deaths from CHD in men and 47 per cent of deaths in women are owing to raised blood cholesterol. Overall, though not for every indicator, the Scots have a poorer set of environmental health inputs than the English.[22]

## Revascularisation Rates[23]

There are two main operations to treat heart disease: coronary artery bypass surgery (CABG) and percutaneous transluminal angioplasty (PTCA). Both are forms of revascularisation. CABG was introduced around 35 years ago, and involves the bypass of a diseased coronary artery using a blood vessel from elsewhere in the body (initially veins from the leg, but increasingly arteries are being used as these have been demonstrated to have greater efficacy). Angioplasty is a more recent invention and involves the insertion of a balloon into the diseased artery to dilate it and increase the blood flow. Advances in technology have meant that increasingly operations that would have been carried out as CABGs are now being carried out as PTCAs. Since 1998 the number of all PTCAs undertaken in the UK has outstripped the number of CABGs. The trend in the

UK, as in nearly all other western European countries, is for an increasing ratio of PTCA to CABG.

Although PTCA rates are slightly higher in England, the number of both procedures has increased dramatically over the last decade in both England and Scotland (see Table 5.1.7). The rate of PTCA and CABG combined per million population is higher in Scotland than in England (Tables 5.1.8 and 5.1.9). The rate of increase has been approximately the same for both countries (between 2000 and 2001, for example, the increase in the number of PTCAs was 17 per cent for Scotland and 16 per cent for England).[24] In spite of these fairly dramatic increases, both Scotland and England lag well behind other western European countries. The OECD ARD team's findings, which relate to the UK rather than Scotland and England, are fairly damning of CHD treatment patterns. Although between 1996 and 2000 the number of PTCAs, for example, increased by 64 per cent in the UK, compared to 40 per cent in France and Switzerland and 44 per cent in Germany, numerically they remain significantly lower. This is in spite of the fact that the UK has greater incidence and mortality from CHD, which suggests greater revascularisation need. According to BCIS data, the rate of PTCA in 2000 was 618 operations per million population in Scotland, 574 in England and 590 in the UK overall.[25] For the same operation the rate in Switzerland was 1,539, in France it was 1,532 and in Germany 2,226. This may in part reflect procedural tendencies in other countries, including some oversupply of healthcare often found in private and social insurance systems,[26] but the total revascularisation rate still reflects significant disparities: the revascularisation rate for the same year was 1,132 per million population in the UK as a whole, compared to 1,815 in France, 2,176 in Switzerland and 3,175 in Germany. It is estimated that at the current rate of growth in coronary interventions, it will take at least ten years before the UK approaches the rates of Switzerland or France.[27]

## Table 5.1.7 : Revascularisation rates

| | 1994 | 1995 | 1996 | 1997 | 1998 | 1999 | 2000 | 2001 | 2002 |
|---|---|---|---|---|---|---|---|---|---|
| **Total revasc.*** | | | | | | | | | |
| Scotland | 3,240 | 3,403 | 3,967 | 4,118 | 4,238 | 4,742 | 4,841 | 4,912 | 5,219 |
| England | 28,550 | 32,317 | N/A | N/A | N/A | 37,202 | 39,321 | 43,834 | 48,679 |
| **Rate per million** | | | | | | | | | |
| Scotland | 635 | 667 | 779 | 810 | 835 | 935 | 956 | 970 | 1,032 |
| England | 593 | 669 | N/A | N/A | N/A | 762 | 803 | 892 | 987 |

*Source*: ISD Scotland; Hospital Episode Statistics

* For the purposes of this study, revascularisation rates will be taken to be the total number of PTCAs and CABGs undertaken as principal operation in a year.

## Table 5.1.8 : CABG rates[28]

| | 1994 | 1995 | 1996* | 1997* | 1998* | 1999 | 2000 | 2001 | 2002 |
|---|---|---|---|---|---|---|---|---|---|
| **Total CABG** | | | | | | | | | |
| Scotland | 2,380 | 2,452 | 2,707 | 2,719 | 2,701 | 2,719 | 2,702 | 2,593 | 2,660 |
| England | 19,564 | 22,192 | N/A | N/A | N/A- | 22,494 | 22,033 | 23,181 | 23,364 |
| **Rate per million‡** | | | | | | | | | |
| Scotland | 466 | 480 | 532 | 535 | 532 | 536 | 534 | 512 | 526 |
| England | 406 | 460 | N/A | N/A | N/A | 461 | 450 | 472 | 474 |

*Source*: ISD Scotland; Hospital Episode Statistics

* Data for 1996-1998 currently unavailable due to transition in HES data provider

‡ Based on mid-year population estimates. Source: ONS, GRO (2002 based on population projection – source: Government Actuary'sDepartment)

### Table 5.1.9
### PTCA rates

| | 1994 | 1995 | 1996 | 1997 | 1998 | 1999 | 2000 | 2001 | 2002 |
|---|---|---|---|---|---|---|---|---|---|
| Total PTCA[†] | | | | | | | | | |
| Scotland | 860 | 951 | 1,260 | 1,399 | 1,537 | 2,023 | 2,139 | 2,319 | 2,559 |
| England | 8,986 | 10,125 | N/A | N/A- | N/A | 14,708 | 17,288 | 20,653 | 25,315 |
| Rate per million | | | | | | | | | |
| Scotland | 169 | 186 | 247 | 275 | 303 | 399 | 422 | 458 | 506 |
| England | 187 | 210 | N/A | N/A | N/A | 301 | 353 | 420 | 513 |

*Source*: ISD Scotland; Hospital Episode Statistics
† OPCS4 codes (principal position) – K49

### Table 5.1.10
### *Certified cardiologists per million population, 1997 and 2000, selected European countries*

| Country | 1997 | 2000 |
|---|---|---|
| France | 83 | 65 |
| Switzerland | 52 | 53 |
| Germany | 24 | 26 |
| UK | 8 | 12 |

*Source*: Block *et al.*, 2003.

*Resources/Facilities*

There has been an acknowledged shortage of specialist staff, from nurses and technicians to cardiac surgeons, in both England and Scotland. In European comparisons the UK fares particularly badly[29] (see Table 5.1.10). In 2000 the UK had only 12 certified cardiologists per million population, compared to 26 in Germany and 65 in France. Overall it had the second-lowest staffing level behind Ireland. This massive gap may in many ways be due to the classification of a 'certified' cardiologists and the standards of qualification, but even if one excludes the outliers such as Greece and Italy (Greece has 240 cardiologists pmp), the EU average is still 43 per million population. Scotland has approximately 70 cardiologists, equating to one for every 73,000 people. England has one cardiologist for every 80,000 people (see Table 5.1.11). The British Cardiac Society recommend a staffing level of one per 70,000 and the 'Fifth report on the provision of services for patients with heart disease' recommends an increase in the number of consultant cardiologists to one per 50,000 in the next four to five years.[30] This equates to an extra 30 consultant cardiologists in Scotland and another 390 in England.

This has been recognised, however, and both the NSF in England and the Coronary Heart Disease and Stroke Strategy for Scotland make provision for an increase in trained staff, and consequently this is a rapidly changing area. The numbers of consultant cardiologists are increasing fairly dramatically in both countries, but there has been a perceptible step-change in recruitment in England. Between 1999 and 2002 the number of consultant cardiologists increased 12.5 per cent in Scotland and 26 per cent in England.

According to the latest available figures,[31] there are currently 33 NHS facilities providing coronary interventions (PTCA's) in England compared to five in Scotland.[32] This equates to around one for every 1.49 million people in England and one for every 1.01 million people in Scotland. There are 31 NHS centres undertaking cardiac surgery (CABG) in England, and four in Scotland.[33]

## Table 5.1.11
### Consultant cardiologists in Scotland and England, 1995-2002

| | | | | | Year | | | |
|---|---|---|---|---|---|---|---|---|
| | 1995 | 1996 | 1997 | 1998 | 1999 | 2000 | 2001 | 2002 |
| **SCOTLAND** | | | | | | | | |
| Headcount | 53 | 60 | 61 | 65 | 66 | 72 | 74 | 74 |
| WTE* | 50 | 58.3 | 59 | 62.6 | 63.4 | 69.3 | 70.3 | 70.4 |
| Consultant:popn (total) | 96,296 | 84,869 | 83,333 | 78,108 | 76,847 | 70,318 | 68,403 | 68,337 |
| Consultant:popn (WTE) | 102,073 | 87,344 | 86,158 | 81,103 | 79,999 | 73,058 | 72,005 | 71,832 |
| **ENGLAND** | | | | | | | | |
| Headcount | 392 | 388 | 405 | 458 | 467 | 546 | 576 | 590 |
| WTE | 351.3 | 349 | 364.3 | 415.4 | 424.6 | 482.1 | 512.1 | N/A |
| Consultant:popn (total) | 123,188 | 124,747 | 119,809 | 106,239 | 104,574 | 89,738 | 85,310 | 83,630 |
| Consultant:popn (WTE) | 137,460 | 138,687 | 133,195 | 117,134 | 115,017 | 101,633 | 95,955 | N/A |

*Source:* ISD Scotland Workforce Statistics; DoH Medical and Dental Workforce Statistics

*Whole-time equivalent (wte) gives a more accurate indication of provision of cardiac staffing as it takes into account part-time work, for cardiologists with academic posts, senior general medical responsibilities etc.

*Preventive treatment*

Prevention of CHD takes two forms: primary prevention (the prevention of CHD in patients who do not as yet manifest any evidence of the condition) and secondary prevention (the prevention of further CHD problems in patients in whom there is already clinical evidence of CHD). There is evidence in both countries of primary prevention being recognised as a major factor in treating CHD. Both the NSF and the CHD & Stroke Strategy for Scotland incorporate primary prevention initiatives. Many of these concern population-based campaigns, such as healthy eating strategies, anti-smoking campaigns and CHD public awareness programmes,[34] evaluation of which would be beyond the remit of this report, but a number of guidelines and recommendations have also been produced for prevention in primary care, the implementation of which can be more easily measured.

*Screening*

There appears to be a general consensus that identification and treatment of those at risk is the key to successful primary prevention. The first priority set out by the NSF is secondary prevention, the reduction of risk in patients who already have coronary heart disease. Standard 3 states: 'General Practitioners and primary care teams should identify all people with established cardiovascular disease and offer them comprehensive advice and appropriate treatment to reduce their risks.' The second priority is identification of high risk patients, set out in Standard 4: 'General practitioners and primary healthcare teams should identify all people at significant risk of cardiovascular disease but who have not yet developed symptoms and offer them appropriate advice and treatment to reduce their risks.' With regard to primary prevention, a high-risk patient is one with an absolute CHD risk of more than 30 per cent over ten years. Risk is calculated by evaluating risk factors such as gender, diabetic status, smoking, age, obesity, hypertension and high cholesterol according to the Joint British Societies Coronary Risk Prediction Chart.

Obviously, emphasis on primary prevention implies some form of screening to identify those at risk. While there is some controversy as to the extent of screening demanded by the NSF,[35] whole-population blood cholesterol concentration monitoring and hypertension monitoring has been dismissed, certainly by the Scottish CHD task force, as an effective primary prevention measure,[36] and so it might well prove fruitless to use the extent of monitoring as a indicator of primary prevention. No provision is made for national screening in the NSF either; the emphasis is rather on opportunistic screening to identify those at greatest risk, and appropriate intervention.

*Action taken on blood pressure (eg for angina – if systolic pressure > 160 mm Hg, or systolic pressure > 140 mm Hg and cholesterol > 5.5 mmol / 1*

No significant data have been collected on this.

*Statin prescription levels*

There is now widespread agreement in both England and Scotland that the use of statins, or other lipid-lowering drugs, is a clinically effective method of reducing the risks of heart disease.[37] The Coronary Heart Disease and Stroke task force report states: 'The evidence of benefit of therapeutic intervention with beta-blockers, ACE inhibitors, aspirins and statins is irrefutable.'[38] Budgetary constraints may play a part in the provision of these drugs, however, as statins are expensive. Table 5.1.12 shows that the level of statin prescription has increased markedly in both Scotland and England. Since 1998 Scotland has had a higher per capita prescription level than England. This is as might be expected, given that prescription levels are generally higher in Scotland by a significant margin. Between 1998 and 2002 prescriptions for statins rose approximately 130 per cent in England, compared to an increase in Scotland for the same time period of around 120 per cent. These are both huge leaps in the use of preventative treatments, and there is some indication that England is gradually gaining on

Scotland. The difference between levels of per capita spending on prescriptions was 29 per cent in 1998 and 25 per cent in 2001. This may in part reflect the step-change generated by the introduction of the National Service Framework in England.

## Table 5.1.12
### Statin prescription levels,[†] England and Scotland, 1998-2002

|  | 1998 | 1999 | 2000 | 2001 | 2002 |
|---|---|---|---|---|---|
| **England** | | | | | |
| No. prescription items (000) | 5,981.50 | 7,925.70 | 10,330.80 | 13,523.00 | 18,800.00* |
| Actual cost[‡] (£000) | 189,966.60 | 256,435.90 | 326,110.50 | 438,845.00 | 546,400.00 |
| Expenditure per capita (£) | 3.90 | 5.25 | 6.65 | 8.93 | 11.07 |
| **Scotland** | | | | | |
| No. prescription items (000) | 786.591 | 1035.20 | 1306.758 | 1592.139 | 1625.123 |
| Actual cost (£000) | 25,538.728 | 34,725.879 | 43,991.437 | 56,313.938 | 70,449.404 |
| Expenditure per capita | 5.03 | 6.85 | 8.69 | 11.12 | 13.93 |

*Source:* ISD Scotland; DoH PCA

† BNF Chapter 2.12. This includes other lipid-lowering drugs, but statins make up 93-96 per cent of the total prescriptions.
‡ In England this is measured as net ingredient cost (NIC); the equivalent in Scotland is gross ingredient cost (GIC).
* Projected full year figures are based on the assumption that statin cost and volume will grow at 30 per cent.
Source: ePACT, Prescription Pricing Authority (PPA).

## 5.2 Stroke Outcomes and Treatment

### Stoke disease statistics we aimed to gather

- Stroke disability and mortality rates

- Number of specialists in stroke medicine

- Specialist stroke units (SSUs) per million

- Rate of use of specialist units in the treatment of stroke patients

- Proportion of health expenditure on stroke treatment

Ten per cent of the world's population died from strokes in 1999, and the WHO in 2000 estimated that between three and eleven per cent of the total disease burden (death and disability) is attributable to stroke. Stroke is the third biggest cause of death in Europe (behind CHD and cancer) and the primary cause of disability.[39] In this respect stroke is something of a hidden health burden, as its costs are borne not only by hospital staff, but also by personal and social services who have to care for those who survive with serious disability. The cost to the NHS of strokes in 1995-6 was estimated to be 4-6 per cent of its total budget.[40]

Considerable variation has been identified in the rates of incidence and stroke mortality across Europe in people under 65, a group in whom stroke is seen as avoidable. The current prevalence rate in the UK is estimated to be five to eight per 1,000 in people over the age of 25. By a number of measures the UK often compares badly with similar European countries such as France and Switzerland.[41] While stroke epidemiology is not as thoroughly understood as that of other diseases, for example CHD, much of the focus of current thinking is on how far the difference in stroke outcome between countries can be attributed to the variable nature of stroke care in those countries. Unfortunately, very few studies have been undertaken comparing stroke trends and treatment in the countries of the UK, and data on stroke incidence, case fatality and in-hospital mortality in Scotland and England, for example, are sparse.

*Stroke Incidence, Mortality and Disability*

*Mortality*

Age-specific mortality from stroke has been declining in both England and Scotland throughout the latter part of the twentieth century[42] (Table 5.2.1), as it has in most other Western European countries.[43] Due to a lack of firm data on trends in stroke incidence and case fatality, no conclusive evidence has yet been presented to account for this decline. Data from comparable international studies on incidence present mixed results, some indicating an overall decline in incidence, some suggesting an increase in incidence in certain groups.[44] More consistent trends appear in studies of case fatality, which appears to have declined internationally (see below). Wade *et al.* argue that the most plausible explanation for the decline in mortality is that both incidence and case fatality have declined, i.e. that improved life-styles and socio-economic factors have lead to diminished risk and also that care has improved, meaning fewer people actually die from stroke. Finding directly comparable data on stroke mortality in the UK is made highly problematic by the way the data are collected and presented in the individual countries.[45] For example, data in England and Northern Ireland are adjusted to European standard population, whereas in Scotland it remains unadjusted. The data reproduced here are from ONS *Regional Trends* surveys and suggest a higher mortality rate in Scotland compared to England, particularly in women. Internationally, the UK as a whole compares more favourably for stroke than it does for coronary heart disease (Table 5.2.2). Between 1990 and 1994 the UK had a higher mortality rate from stroke than France and Switzerland but a lower mortality rate than Germany, Austria, Spain and Italy.[46] In 2002, using World Health Organisation data (WHOSIS) for 17 countries, Leon *et al.* found that Scotland's rank position has fluctuated between second and third place over the past 40 years in both men and women.[47]

## Table 5.2.1

*Mortality from cerebrovascular disease, per 100,000, England and Scotland, 1993-1999\**

| | | | | | Death rate per 100,000 | | |
| --- | --- | --- | --- | --- | --- | --- | --- |
| | 1993 | 1994 | 1995 | 1996 | 1997 | 1998 | 1999 |
| **Men** | | | | | | | |
| Scotland | 129 | 123 | 116 | 109 | 106 | 103 | 99 |
| England | 98 | 84 | 81 | 80 | 77 | 75 | 71 |
| UK | 101 | 88 | 84 | 83 | 80 | 78 | 74 |
| **Women** | | | | | | | |
| Scotland | 164 | 203 | 197 | 177 | 171 | 170 | 169 |
| England | 155 | 138 | 133 | 133 | 127 | 125 | 123 |
| UK | 160 | 144 | 140 | 138 | 132 | 130 | 127 |
| **All** | | | | | | | |
| Scotland | N/A | 163 | 157 | 144 | 139 | 137 | 135 |
| England | N/A | 112 | 108 | 107 | 103 | 101 | 98 |
| UK | N/A | 117 | 112 | 111 | 107 | 104 | 101 |

*Source*: ONS *Regional Trends* 30-37

\* Stroke ICD9 430-438, ICD10 160-169 (coding system changed 1999)

## Table 5.2.2

### Cerebrovascular disease mortality, ranking and number of neurologists

| Country | Italy | Denmark | France | Germany | Hungary | Netherlands | CH | UK | USA |
|---|---|---|---|---|---|---|---|---|---|
| Cerebrovascular mortality per 100,000 (a) | | | | | | | | | |
| Male | N/A | 66.0 | 48.5 | 70.7 | 178.9 | 61.6 | 54.3 | 66.8 | 44.7 |
| (b) | N/A | (5) | (2) | (7) | (8) | (4) | (3) | (6) | (1) |
| Female | N/A | 51.8 | 34.5 | 54.4 | 119.7 | 51.4 | 41.3 | 61.1 | 40.9 |
| | N/A | (5) | (1) | (6) | (8) | (4) | (3) | (7) | (2) |
| Number of neurologists | 10.4 | 4.6 | N/A | N/A | 0.4 | 4+ | N/A | 0.4 | N/A |

Mortality information is from OECD Health Data 2002. Neurologist figures are from OECD, ARD team (2002).
(a) 1997 figures standardised to the European standard population, aged 40 and over.
(b) numbers in parenthesis are rankings.

*Incidence*

Owing to the way in which incidence statistics are gathered in England, it is not a straightforward task to measure incidence rate from hospital episodes.[48] However a number of studies have been undertaken into cases of first-ever stroke in England. [49] Using the results from these, and data from English health surveys, it is possible to estimate a rate of incidence for England. It has been estimated that stroke rate incidence is between 174 and 216 per 100,000 population for the year 2000. For Scotland, using hospital-based reporting, the incidence rate has been estimated at 230 per hundred thousand.[50] While these data preclude any certain conclusions, due to the considerable methodological differences in collection, a study published in May 2003 indicated that Scotland has a far higher incidence rate than England, in fact one of the highest incidence rates in the World.[51] However age-adjusted incidence rates proved similar to other population-based studies—indicating that the high crude rate was due to an older survey population.

Table 5.2.3 shows the prevalence of stroke as reported in health surveys for England and Scotland. The prevalence of stroke has been estimated at 220 per 100,000 population for women and 330 per 100,000 population for men, aged 55 to 64. This compares with 260 women per 100,000 population and 210 men per 100,000 population for the same age cohort in Scotland.[52]

Any conclusions on comparative incidence and prevalence are difficult to draw due to a lack of current evidence, although, excluding the data for men from the Joint Health Surveys, it would appear that generally Scotland has a higher incidence of stroke. Certainly, it would be implausible to account for the far higher mortality rates in Scotland compared to England simply by differences in care alone. In international comparisons of stroke incidence, for which comparable data for England only have been collected, it would appear that England has a higher incidence of stroke than France, but lower incidence than Germany.[53] The OECD ARD team found that Sweden, Norway, Italy and Denmark have the highest incidence rates among the countries studied, while the UK and Australia have the lowest incidence.[54]

*Table 5.2.3*
*Percentage who have experienced stroke*
*(ever and currently), England and Scotland, 1998*

|  |  | Age | | |
|---|---|---|---|---|
|  |  | 45-54 | 55-64 | 65-75 |
|  |  | % | % | % |
| **Men** |  |  |  |  |
|  | Currently (b) |  |  |  |
| England |  | 0.2 | 0.8 | 1.4 |
| Scotland |  | 0.5 | 0.0 (a) | 1.2 |
|  | Ever |  |  |  |
| England |  | 1.2 | 3.3 | 6.2 |
| Scotland |  | 0.9 | 2.1 | 6.4 |
| **Women** |  |  |  |  |
|  | Currently |  |  |  |
| England |  | 0.1 | 0.7 | 0.5 |
| Scotland |  | 0.1 | 0.2 | 1.1 |
|  | Ever |  |  |  |
| England |  | 0.7 | 2.2 | 5.0 |
| Scotland |  | 0.5 | 2.6 | 5.5 |

*Source*: Health Survey for England 1998, table 2.1; Scottish Health Survey 1998, table 2.1.
(a) this figure (0.0) is as printed in the source. (b) in the last 12 months

## Stroke risk factors

Smoking and hypertension are the main risk factors for stroke. Others include high cholesterol, being overweight, high alcohol consumption, certain medical conditions, and low socio-economic status.[55]

## Case fatality

Case fatality gives some idea of survival rates from stroke, and as such may be more helpful than mortality and incidence in giving some indication of the nature of stroke care. There are a number of pan-European studies of stroke survival (BIOMED, EROS, MONICA, IST) although the data representing the UK are nearly all from England. Again, there is little data that will allow a comparison of case fatality in England compared to Scotland. We can use international comparisons instead, however, and using the conclusions they make between stroke outcomes and healthcare inputs, take what we do know about stroke provision in England and Scotland, to make tentative conclusions about how the two might compare.

In all studies the UK was shown to have consistently worse outcomes than similar European countries. Wolfe *et al.* showed that three-month fatality rates in UK (English) centres varied from 31 per cent to 39 per cent compared to 20 per cent in France, and 28 per cent in Italy. Case fatality in Germany varied between 19 per cent and 27 per cent.[56] The EROS study showed that the case fatality rate was again highest in the UK, although incidence was in fact lower than in Germany. (Incidence was found to be 123.9 per 100,000 in London, compared to 136.4 per 100,000 in Erlangen, while case fatality was 41 per cent compared to 34 per cent.)[57] The International Stroke Trial demonstrated that the difference in the proportion of patients dead or dependent in the UK and other countries was between 150 and 300 events per 1,000.[58] There is considerable speculation as to what extent these differences can be attributed to differences in stroke care, particularly in the acute phase. It is difficult to establish any clear causal relations to account for the difference in outcome, particularly the impact of stroke care. The major factor often not controlled for is severity of stroke, which may well vary across countries and over time. Furthermore, the International Stroke Trial found that differences in outcome between the UK and other countries are 'much larger than might plausibly be explained by differential use of even the most efficacious of known interventions'. While they establish no clear causal relations to explain difference in case fatality, Wolfe *et al.* did note consistently low intervention rates for controlling abnormal physiology in the acute phase of stroke in the UK. Likewise, the International Stroke Trial noted that in Scandanavian countries—among the earliest advocates of the organisation and specialisation of stroke care—some of the lowest case fatality rates were found. However, mortality rates do not reflect incidence (see Tables 5.2.2-5.2.4).

The OECD ARD team recorded in-hospital mortality and one-year case mortality.[59] The eleven countries studied were put into one of three groups: a low death rate, medium death rate or a high death rate. Only the UK is classified as high.[60] In-hospital mortality reveals few differences between countries, with the exception of the UK which has significantly higher fatality rates in the first seven days for all age-groups. Fatalities in the UK were roughly twice the average. About nine per cent of those aged 4-64 were dead within a week of arriving in hospital. In other countries the figure was around five per cent.[61] The OECD also compared death rates after one year in order to reflect the care provided by GPs as well as the hospitals. According to the ARD team, the UK falls outside the normal ranges. For example, in the USA 37 per cent of stroke victims aged 75 or more were dead within a year, but in the UK it was 57 per cent. These figures should be interpreted with caution, as the severity of cases admitted was not controlled for, and there are different admission practices between countries. However, case fatality rates include care outside hospital and a similar pattern is seen to that for in-hospital mortality. Rates are lowest in Denmark, and highest by far in the UK, suggesting that the standard of care in the UK is inadequate.

*Table 5.2.4*
*Hospital and case fatality rates*
*for ischaemic stroke patients*

| | |
|---|---|
| Low fatality rates | Denmark, Sweden, Switzerland, Japan |
| Medium fatality rates | Norway, US, Australia, Canada, Italy, Spain |
| High fatality rates | UK |

Source: derived from OECD, ARD team (2002). p. 19.

## Specialist Stroke Units: provision and rate of use

It is now broadly accepted that organised stroke services (specialist stroke units) can considerably reduce the risk of disability or death from stroke,[62] some studies indicating that this reduction may be as much as 25 per cent.[63] No unified definition of a 'stroke unit' exists; dedicated stroke services in hospitals across the UK can range from geographically defined areas in hospitals dealing with acute and rehabilitative procedures, to teams dealing with rehabilitation alone. The types of 'stroke unit' that have been identified are presented below:[64]

- stroke ward: geographically defined area where stroke patients receive stroke unit care

- stroke team: a mobile team delivering stroke unit care to patients in a variety of wards; this does not always include a specialist nurse

- dedicated stroke unit: a disease-specific stroke unit managing only stroke patients

- mixed assessment/rehabilitation unit: a generic disability unit (which fulfils the definition of a stroke unit) specialising in the management of disabling illnesses including stroke; for example, this would include geriatric and neurological rehabilitation wards

- acute stroke unit: a stroke unit accepting patients acutely and continuing for several days (usually <1 week)

- combined acute/rehabilitation stroke unit: a stroke unit accepting patients acutely but continuing care for several weeks if necessary

- rehabilitation stroke unit: a stroke unit accepting patients after a delay of one to two weeks and continuing care for several weeks if necessary.

The paucity of well-organised stroke care and inconsistency of stroke provision in the UK has long been acknowledged within the medical profession.[65] Patients suffering from stroke are often more likely than those in other European countries to be treated in a general medical ward or elderly care unit that does not meet the criteria of organised stroke care.[66] This may well contribute to worse stroke outcomes (see above). When the OECD collected specialist stroke unit information for four countries, in

Sweden 70 per cent of stroke patients were cared for in a specialist unit, in Norway 60 per cent, in the UK 26 per cent and in Hungary 15 per cent.[67] However, the inadequacy of stroke provision, in addition to poor stroke outcomes across the UK generally, has been recognised in recent years, and this has lead to considerable development of strategic stroke provision. The NHS in Scotland has produced a combined coronary heart disease and stroke strategy, which includes provision for 1,000 more designated stroke beds. In England, Standard 5 of the National Service Framework for Older People is devoted to stroke care. Consequently the data presented here might not quite reflect the current situation, as it is rapidly changing. Using data from the Stroke Association Survey of 1998, provision of specialised stroke services can be illustrated as follows in Tables 5.2.5 and 5.2.6.

### Table 5.2.5
### Total number of SSUs, England and Scotland, 1998

|          | Acute only | Rehabilitation Only | Acute/ Rehabilitation | Team (no unit) | All forms of SSU |
|----------|------------|---------------------|-----------------------|----------------|------------------|
| England  | 21         | 93                  | 19                    | 3              | 136              |
| Scotland | 9          | 16                  | 4                     | N/A            | 29               |

Source: Ebrahim 1999

### Table 5.2.6
### SSUs per million population, England and Scotland, 1998*

|          | Acute only | Rehabilitation Only | Acute/ Rehabilitation | Team (no unit) | All forms of SSU |
|----------|------------|---------------------|-----------------------|----------------|------------------|
| England  | 0.43       | 1.91                | 0.39                  | 0.06           | 2.80             |
| Scotland | 1.77       | 3.15                | 0.79                  | N/A            | 5.71             |

Source: Ebrahim 1999

* Assuming Scottish population at 30 June 1998 5, 077,070; English population 48,657,500. Source: GRO Scotland; ONS England and Wales.

It is clear, then, that the cover for stroke care is much better in Scotland than in England, although stroke provision is progressing rapidly. According to the latest available figures, there are now 175 sites in England, Wales and Northern Ireland providing specialised stroke services.[68] In Scotland 33 hospitals admit patients at the acute stage and others take patients for rehabilitation after acute discharge.[69]

More important than the provision of stroke units is access to those units. Across the UK, at best half of all patients admitted in 1998 were managed by an organised stroke service. Within the UK there is considerable variation. Perhaps significantly, the survey showed that patients admitted to hospitals in Scotland were twice as likely to be admitted to an SSU than those in England. The percentage of patients admitted or transferred to a stroke unit was 65 per cent in Scotland, compared to an average of 49 per cent in England. (However, there was considerable regional variation with admission rates in Trent reaching those in Scotland and those in the South West nearly half of those in Scotland.) Later figures from the 2001/2 *National Sentinel Stroke Audit* reveal that, although 73 per cent of sites have a stroke unit, only 36 per cent of admitted patients spend any time on a stroke unit and only 27 per cent spend the majority of their stay on the unit. Similar current figures for Scotland are not available. Further data on acute treatment of stroke victims seem to indicate a similar level of treatment in both countries. In Scotland patients underwent acute stage timely dysphagia screening in only 52 per cent of trusts in 1998.[70] In England for the same year this figure was 55 per cent.[71]

*Specialists in stroke medicine*

The availability of specialists has a significant impact on outcomes and the UK has a significantly smaller number per 100,000 population (the number of neurologists per 100,000 is shown in Table 5.2.2).[72] However, assessing the level of stroke specialist staffing is often difficult, as there is disagreement as to the definition of a stroke specialist. Some data are available, however. In England, Wales and Northern Ireland, 80 per cent of trusts have a consultant physician with specialist knowledge of stroke formally recognised as having principal responsibility for stroke services.[73] This compares to 64 per cent in 1998. In Scotland 71 per cent of hospitals providing stroke care have an acute consultant, and 82 per cent have a rehabilitation consultant.[74] Levels of staffing, therefore, are fairly even between the two countries. There appear to have been significant improvements in the provision of organised stroke care in both countries, but more research is required to identify where these improvements are progressing faster.

## 5.3 Cancer Outcomes and Treatment[75]

- Cancer Treatment Recent Development in the UK
- English Cancer Care Architecture
- Scottish Cancer Care Architecture
- Incidence and Outcomes
- Cancer Treatment

*Cancer statistics we attempted to gather:*

- Number of specialist radiologists
- Number of palliative care specialists (breast, lung, colon, etc) per patient
- Specialist cancer units for each cancer
- Breast cancer—prevalence of breast-conserving therapy, breast-conserving therapy with post-operative radiation therapy, and mastectomy (include rates by age-group). Rates of surgical resection for stage I or II non-small cell lung cancer
- Access to radiation therapy
- Use of taxanes

### Cancer Treatment Development in the UK

International opinion on ideal cancer treatment methods has changed in recent years. In 1995, the EUROCARE study reported that some specialists seemed to do better than generalists.[76] Additionally, specialists treating a larger number of patients tend to have better results. Evidence from ovarian, breast, oesophagus, stomach, testis and sarcoma cancers exists to support this idea;[77] 'when cancer of the breast was studied, it seemed that surgeons who specialise in the condition could obtain 17 per cent better survival.' Further evidence suggests that treatment in specialised centres with a multidisciplinary approach leads to improved outcomes.[78]

This evidence pre-dates the UK's well-known Expert Advisory Group on Cancer (Calman-Hine) Report of 1995, which set out seven principles to govern cancer care (see annex), and recommended the creation of cancer centres and cancer units with experts in cancer working collaboratively in multidisciplinary teams. Calman-Hine envisaged that cancer centres serving populations over one million would be sited in large general hospitals providing radiotherapy and sophisticated diagnostic technology (MRI, CT scanning) for the region. Cancer units, charged with integrating primary and secondary care, and looking after the more common cancers, would be found in district hospitals. Both units and centres would have surgical subspecialisation.[79] The Calman-Hine recommendations, which were welcomed by all, have been likened to an oncological McDonalds: standardised and with failsafe quality control.[80]

In 1999, Professor Karol Sikora described the implementation of Calman-Hine as a 'saga of under-resourcing and bureaucratic muddle'.[81] A major problem has been 'the lack of new resources to implement change'.[82] Before we present some outcomes data, it is important that we set out recent reforms in cancer treatment architecture in Scotland and England.

### *English Cancer Care Architecture*

The *Health of the Nation* strategy for England in 1992 identified cancer as one of five key areas in which improvement was required; cancers of the lung, breast and cervix being singled out for special attention.[83] Some years later in *Saving Lives: Our Healthier Nation* the Government reported that overall death rates from cancer in England for people under 65 are slightly better than the EU average, but went on to say that this figure conceals some important differences. The UK death rates from breast and cervical cancer are some of the worst in Europe.[84] In this context, *Our Healthier Nation* set a target: 'to reduce the death rate from cancer amongst people aged under 65 years by at least a further fifth by 2010'. A National Cancer Director / Tsar, Professor Mike Richards, was appointed in 2000 to oversee the improvement of English cancer care.

*The NHS Cancer Plan (Referral and Treatment Guidelines)*

The Cancer Plan forms part of the framework to tackle cancer mortality in England; it acknowledges that patients in England often have poorer survival rates than those in other European countries. It suggests that for a number of cancers such as breast and bowel, poor survival may be due to delay in diagnosis—with the result that the disease is at a more advanced stage by the time treatment commences. The Plan's aim is to reduce death rates by 20 per cent by 2010, largely by a set of ambitious targets on waiting and referral times. It stated that, for all cancers by 2005, there will be a maximum one-month wait from diagnosis to initiation of treatment.[85] Note that in 2000 the Government pledged that patients with suspected cancer would have a two-week maximum wait for referral from GP to specialist.[86] The Cancer Plan also embraced many of Calman-Hine's other recommendations, including the introduction of cancer centres and units working in cancer networks, and greater specialisation in cancer care.[87] Nevertheless, geographical variation in cancer treatment was still significant. To ensure that patients across England receive the same standard of care, by March 2002 treatment guidelines for a range of cancers had been issued.

*Cancer registries*

Cancer registration in the parts of the UK began in 1929 and achieved national coverage in 1962.[88] Nine regional cancer registries have been collecting cancer data since then. Their main priority is to guarantee a uniform process of registering cancers region-wide, so that comparable data can be sent to the ONS and in some cases to international publications (such as EUROCARE).

*Cancer networks and the Cancer Services Collaborative*

First envisaged in Calman-Hine, there are now 34 local cancer networks in England each covering a population of roughly 1.5 million. The networks reach from primary care to specialist cancer units and thus bring together health service commissioners and providers. Each network works closely with PCT cancer leads. PCT leads are a joint initiative between the Department of Health and Macmillan Cancer Relief to invest £5,000 per PCT (since April 2001) to enable 'the lead clinician to have dedicated time to contribute to the development of cancer networks and raising the standard of care within the PCT'.[89]

The NHS Cancer Plan announced: 'To help cancer networks reshape the services they provide to ensure fast, efficient, streamlined care, the new NHS Modernisation Agency will lead the roll out of the Cancer Services Collaborative (CSC) to all cancer networks by 2002. Part of the Modernisation Agency, the CSC is an NHS programme charged with improving 'the experience and outcomes for patients with suspected or diagnosed cancer by optimising care delivery systems across the whole pathway of care'. Specifically, it guides providers through the 34 cancer networks and 600 teams,[90] in the delivery of improvement targets set out in the Cancer Plan.

*Reducing cancer incidence*

Writing in the *BMJ* in early 2003, Susan Mayor noted that cancer care in the UK has been improving, primarily because there have been successes in reducing cancer incidence, for example by significant reductions in numbers of those who smoke.[91] Cutting tobacco consumption has been a key aim (see NHS Cancer Plan); cessation services have been established throughout the country and around 250,000 people have stopped smoking since April 2000; the government's target is 1.5 million by 2010.[92] A number of other lifestyle factors such as diet, alcohol consumption and level of exercise are linked to cancer incidence. The NHS Cancer Plan (Chapter 2) includes targets for these too.

*Cancer resources*

In 1991 the Royal College of Radiologists reported that there were too few oncologists in the UK and that their workload was too high.[93] Ten years on, the present Government's cancer plans are heavily dependent on the recruitment of thousands more health professionals. Ministers planned to recruit 1,000 extra specialist oncologists by 2006 but, as Karol Sikora noted, a major problem has been 'the lack of new resources to implement change'.[94] That was in 1999, so have the significant resources pumped into the NHS since then led to change? In 2002, the OECD's ARD team criticised the UK's poor breast cancer performance. By early 2003, the Annual Report of the NHS Modernisation Board suggests some progress, but the 'the lack of trained staff remains the biggest single problem' and as a result the cancer workforce works under great pressure. The report continues: 'We particularly need more doctors, nurses, radiographers, biomedical scientists and administrative support staff.'[95] Despite extra resources being pumped into cancer care, there are real concerns that money is not reaching the frontline.

*Breast and cervical screening*

The NHS has two national population screening programmes; that for breast cancer (NHSBSP) and for cervical cancer. Screening for breast cancer was introduced in England (and Scotland) in 1988, following the Forrest Committee Report of 1987.[96] There is a national co-ordination office in Sheffield. Women aged 50-64 years are invited for mammography every three years.[97] Following evidence of benefit to those over 64, in 2000 the National Screening Committee recommended that those aged 65-69, should also be invited to screening. This reform was duly announced in the Cancer Plan, and is to be implemented in England by 2004.[98] The Annual Report (2003) of the NHS Modernisation Board acknowledges that this reform is underway; roughly 100,000 more women were invited to be screened in the year to October 2002.[99] The Cancer Plan also undertook that all women screened would have two views of their breasts taken.[100] The budget for the English breast screening programme is approximately £52 million (roughly £30 per woman invited, or £40 per woman screened). Key breast and cervical cancer screening facts may be found below.

*Results*

It is said that cancer services in England have improved since the Calman-Hine Report, but there is still evidence of poor co-ordination.[101] Three years on from his contribution to *Realities of Rationing*, Karol Sikora is still highly critical, and argues that recently trumpeted progress amounts little more than government propaganda.[102] There is also significant geographical variation in cancer incidence, treatment and survival within the UK and within its constituent parts.[103]

In December 2001 a report by the Audit Commission and CHI, published the first in a series of reviews of NSF implementation.[104] The implementation of recent guidelines and the NHS Cancer Plan for England (September 2000) was also assessed. Although professional specialisation is improving, and most trusts now claim to have lists of sub-specialties for all types of cancer, nevertheless the report found that many patients are operated on by non-specialists, even where a specialist is available.[105]

Guidelines on referral times are largely being met—98 per cent of patients with suspected cancer are seen within two weeks of referral.[106] But many with prostate cancer wait longer—up to six weeks.[107] There are also 'serious and unacceptable' delays in obtaining certain tests. For example, the average wait for a bladder endoscopy was 88 days. The report's researchers suggested that this was due to lack of staff (e.g. radiographers and pathologists), shortages of imaging equipment, and underuse of available resources. [108] The ONS reported that the implementation of breast cancer guidelines has been slow.[109] Meanwhile a report published in 2001 by independent advisory group NCEPOD claimed that emergency treatment for cancer patients is poor, even in specialist units, because of a shortage of specialist doctors.[110]

## Scottish Cancer Care Architecture

### Scottish Cancer Group

Having overtaken heart disease as the leading cause of premature death in 1999, cancer is clearly one of the greatest health problems in Scotland.[111] The need to improve cancer care in the light of the increasing prevalence of people living with cancers is acknowledged by the Scottish Executive: by the age of 74 one in four men and women can expect to be diagnosed with cancer.[112] The Scottish Cancer Group (SCG) was established in 1998. The SCG now:

> leads and directs the cancer services reconfiguration programme in Scotland ...[It] is a multi-disciplinary group which advises Ministers, the Chief Medical Officer and the Health Department on the strategic priorities and objectives for the development of cancer services, including service quality, research and audit, clinical trials, and clinical effectiveness. The Group also provides advice on trends in incidence and mortality, scientific advances and on the implementation of nationally agreed initiatives for the delivery of cancer services, programmes of prevention and screening.[113]

The SCG was reformed in summer 2001 to incorporate voluntary sector and patient views.

Early in its work, the SCG determined that Quality Assurance of cancer services was important. Definitive standards were drawn up for four cancers. This was done in collaboration with the Clinical Standards Board for Scotland (CSBS), which became part of the NHS Quality Improvement Scotland (NHSQIS) in January 2003, and which now monitors their implementation. [114]

In order to identify priority areas for action, the SCG commissioned a detailed study, published in 2001 (*Cancer Scenarios*), which set out the likely effects of cancer and planning needs in Scotland over the next decade.[115] The Scottish Executive's Cancer Plan,[116] *Cancer in Scotland:*

*Action for Change*, drew on the lessons presented in *Cancer Scenarios*.[117]

## Referral and treatment guidelines

*Action for Change* contains commitments on referral and subsequent treatment waiting times. For example: 'By October 2001, women who have breast cancer and are referred for urgent treatment will begin that treatment within one month of diagnosis, where clinically appropriate'.[118] There is a general target that by 2005 the maximum wait from urgent referral to treatment for all cancers will be two months. [119]

In the context of commitments in *Action for Change*[120] and the earlier *Our National Health: a plan for action, a plan for change*,[121] April 2002 saw the publication of *Scottish Referral Guidelines for Suspected Cancer*. The guidelines, which are designed to enable GPs to identify patients requiring urgent specialist investigation, were developed by a sub-group of the SCG.[122]

The SCG is responsible for overseeing the implementation of *Action for Change*, which promised £40 million of investment in cancer services over the period 2001-2004.

## Cancer Centres, Cancer Networks and The Cancer Services Collaborative

Scotland has five specialist cancer centres; one in each of the major cities.[123] As in England, and following the Calman-Hine recommendations, *Action for Change*[124] committed NHSScotland to the development by 2002 of 'managed clinical networks' (MCNs)[125] which would bring together 'cancer professionals and organisations from primary, secondary and tertiary care to work in a coordinated manner, transcending geographical, organisational and professional boundaries'.[126] It was estimated that such networks could lead to mortality reductions of between five and ten per cent.[127] There are three MCNs: the North of Scotland Cancer Network (NOSCAN); West of Scotland Network (WOSCAN); and South East Scotland Cancer Network (SCAN). Each of these three networks has established Regional Cancer Advisory Groups (RCAGs) which provide update reports to the SCG. The RCAGs work with the Health Boards to produce local investment plans which are then submitted to the SCG.[128]

*Registration*

National cancer registration in Scotland began in 1959 and, in comparison to other registries, is considered unusual in its completeness and accuracy. Today registration is co-ordinated by the Scottish Cancer Registry of the Scottish Cancer Intelligence Unit (SCIU) at the Information and Statistics Division (ISD) of the NHS in Scotland. The SCIU provides information on the incidence, prevalence and outcome of cancer in Scotland.[129]

*Reducing cancer incidence*

*Cancer in Scotland: Action for Change* acknowledges that the prevention of cancer requires the changing of personal lifestyles—by stopping smoking, eating a better diet and taking more exercise. Public health efforts have been concentrated on these areas for some time; in 2000 the Scottish Executive announced the creation of a new £100 million Health Improvement Fund which was to 'invest the entire Scottish allocation of extra tobacco tax in public health'.[130] The number of Scottish men who smoke has already fallen dramatically, but further targets have been set to reduce the rate of smoking from an average of 35 per cent to 33 per cent between 1995 and 2005, and to 31 per cent by 2010.[131] Nicotine replacement therapy (NRT) products are now available on prescription in order to help more people stop smoking.[132] There are diet, alcohol consumption and exercise targets too. For example, there is a Scottish Executive Plan for Action on Alcohol Problems;[133] and a National Physical Activity Task Force has been established to increase activity among all age-groups.

*Cancer resources*

The five specialist hospital cancer centres provide treatments such as radiotherapy and chemotherapy. Specialist oncologists based in these 'centres travel extensively to provide support and care to patients across the country'.[134] *Action for Change* highlights the fact that increases in demands on radiology and pathology have not been met by parallel increases 'in resources, particularly for staff.'[135] Imaging technology is also in short supply in Scotland. There can be significant delays, in particular for MRI scans (both diagnostic and for follow-up). In addition, and in light of evidence from the USA, the Health Technology Board for Scotland (HTBS—since January 2003 part of NHSQIS), is carrying out a review of Positron Emission Tomography (PET) scanning technology.

According to *Our National Health: A plan for action, a plan for change*, Scotland had 1,200 radiographers in 2000.[136] November 2001 saw the announcement of £10 million extra resources for NHS recruitment that were to result in 28 more cancer specialists as well as extra nurses and radiographers being employed in Scotland.[137]

*Breast and cervical screening*

The Scottish Executive takes into account the advice of the UK National Screening Committee, which was established in 1996 to advise UK health ministers.

The UK breast screening programme was introduced following the recommendations of a working party that found evidence that screening could reduce mortality by up to 30 per cent.[138] The Scottish breast cancer screening programme (SBCSP) began in 1988, aiming to cut mortality by 20 per cent by 2010. It has a target uptake of 70 per cent. The programme invites women aged between 50 and 64 to be screened once every three years. As in England, the upper age limit for the SBCSP is to rise from 65 to 70 years starting in 2003/04. Women over 70 can continue to be screened if they request.[139] There are six static screening centres in Scotland, and 13 mobile units.

The percentage of all those invited to screening who attend in Scotland has increased a little from around 71 per cent to 73 per cent (1990-2001)—though these figures hide significant variation between those at different points of

Carstairs' Deprivation Category: those on the lowest level of the scale had a take up of c. 51 per cent while 78 per cent (1996/7 figures) of those on the top level of the scale attended.[140] There are also significant geographical variations in screening take-up, with high rates seen in Grampian (83 per cent), Shetland (86.9 per cent) and Orkney (88.5 per cent). Low rates are seen in the industrial central belt (Glasgow 66.2 per cent, Lanarkshire 69.3 per cent, Lothian 69.7 per cent).

Cervical screening in Scotland is available to women aged 20-60 every three to five years. Those over 60 can be screened on request. Colorectal[141] and prostate[142] cancer screening pilots are now taking place in Scotland. Evidence suggests that screening could reduce colorectal cancer deaths by c. 15 per cent. In December 2002 the BBC reported favourable results from the first phase of the colorectal screening trial, which is based at Dundee's King's Cross Hospital. It is reported that the Scottish Executive has provided £2.5 million to continue the scheme until a decision on national screening is taken.[143]

## Cancer Incidence and Outcomes

Cancer is one of the major causes of death in the UK. The following sections present cancer incidence, age standardised mortality, and survival for England and Scotland. We also include the results of the EUROCARE II study which, though a little old, put cancer survival in Scotland and England in an international context.

Incidence of cancer is a measure of new cases in a given period; it depends on a number of factors including age, genetic make-up, diet and smoking behaviour. As the incidence of cancer is heavily age-dependent, it is advisable to age-standardise the rates when comparing populations with different age structures. Cancer prevalence is often used in place of incidence; prevalence refers to those diagnosed with cancer who are alive at a given time.[144] Cancer survival is an important indicator of the efficacy of cancer treatment; it is typically measured over one and five years post diagnosis.

## Box 5.3.1
## Cancer survival rates: England vs Scotland*

**England**: Of 72 survival rates:

- *46 were below* the European average
- *5 were > 10 percentage points below* the European average

  Including:    -1 and 5 year survival rates of gastric cancer

  -5 year survival of prostate cancer

  -5 year survival of chronic lymphocyic leukemia

- *13 were above* the European average

  Including:    -5 year survival rates for nasopharyngeal cancer

  -1 and 5 year survival rates of bone cancer

  -5 year survival, gynaecological tumours of cervix uteri

  -5 year survival (ages 15-44) non-Hodgkins lymphoma

  -5 year survival (ages 15-44) Hodgkin's disease

  -1 and 5 year survival of malignant melanoma

- *8 were the same* as the European average

**Scotland**: Of 72 survival rates:

- *48 were below* the European average
- *10 were > 10 percentage points below* the European average

  Including:    -Female 1 and 5 year survival of nasophayngeal cancer

  -1 and 5 year survival of gastric cancer

  -Male 5 year survival of bone cancer

  -5 year survival of kidney cancer

  -5 year survival (ages 15-44) chronic myelocytic leukemia

  -5 year survival (ages 15-44) chronic lymphocytic leukemia

- *9 were above* the European average

  Including    -Male 1 year survival of bone cancer

  -5 year survival from testicular cancer

  -5 year survival of acute lymphoblastic leukemia

  -5 year survival of (ages 15-44) non-Hodgkins lymphoma

  -1 and 5 year survival of malignant melanoma

- *1 was > 10 percentage points above* the European average

  -5 year survival (ages 15-44) acute lymphoblastic leukemia

- *4 were the same* as the European average

*Note*: This summary compares the cancer survival rates from England and Scotland. 28 cancers were surveyed, and 72 survival rates (one- and five-years for males and females) calculated in the course of the EUROCARE II Survey.

The findings of the EUROCARE II study were published in 1999, and have been very widely cited since then. Box 5.3.1 above summarises the EUROCARE II study results for Scotland and England. It shows that both countries performed poorly overall in comparison to other participating countries, usually falling some way behind the EU average for both relative one-year and five-year survival.[145] At least starting from such a low base, arguably owing to decades of under-investment in UK health care, it is likely that rapid improvements in cancer care and survival have been and will continue to be made both in England and Scotland.

A debate on the interpretation and validity of the EUROCARE results has arisen, particularly in the UK; the position of England and Scotland therefore warrants some comment as some consider the data used to be rather unreliable.[146] For example, in 1998 Prior, Woodman and Collins of the University of Manchester Centre for Cancer Epidemiology suggested 'three possible explanations for the five-year advantage enjoyed by the EUROCARE cohort [compared to the Scots and English]: more patients may have been 'cured', a larger proportion of patients with *in situ* disease may have been misclassified as having invasive disease, or a substantial number of cases of advanced disease were not ascertained.' Prior *et al.* argue that we should treat comparisons across populations which 'vary in accuracy and completeness of registration' with caution, as 'differences in outcome may not reflect differences in the quality of care but more effective cancer registration'. Nevertheless the authors acknowledge significant variation in outcomes within the UK, and consider that 'substantial improvements in survival are most likely to follow from a reduction in the number of patients presenting with advanced disease.'[147]

Also casting doubt on EUROCARE's findings, in 2001 Woodman *et al.* suggested that in light of the commitments in the National Cancer Plan, we should compare our cancer outcome performance with Scandinavian countries where complete registration is long established (the Scottish findings regarding incidence and survival have been described as an artefact because data registration is unusually complete). However, Woodman *et al.* acknowledged 'that cancer survival is poorer in the UK than in the countries they consider worthy comparators'.[148] EURO-

CARE authors have responded to their critics. Gatta, Capocaccia, and Berrino consider that Woodman *et al.*'s assertion that UK survival rates should only be compared with those of Finland and Scandinavia is based on prejudice rather than evidence.[149] Replying to a published letter relating to their lung-cancer survival findings, which suggested that 'cancer care might be no worse in the UK than in the rest of Europe,[150] Forman, Gatta, Capocaccia, Janssen-Heijnen, Coebergh write: 'The EUROCARE findings are in accord with what is known about international variation in the use of diagnostic procedures and appropriate therapeutic interventions for lung cancer. Indeed the lower proportion of microscopically verified cases, noted by Cookson, shows that fewer cancer patients receive investigations and surgery in the UK than in other European countries. Cancer survival in European countries can be broadly correlated with the proportion of the gross national product spent on health. There are also differing medical cultural attitudes within the UK about the treatability of certain cancer patients. It is time for some UK doctors to take their heads out of the sand.'[151]

Perhaps it is not safe to draw conclusions about the effectiveness or efficiency of healthcare systems across Europe solely on the basis of EUROCARE cancer data. Nevertheless, for the purposes of this report, the EURO-CARE study shows that, in many cases, Scottish survival rates were slightly worse than those in England. However, Scotland outperforms England for five-year survival in male lung, prostate, melanoma, testicular cancer and female melanoma, colon, and bladder cancer.[152] Late presentation is one important explanation for poor survival rates factor. In 2000, a comprehensive Scottish study (*Trends in Cancer Survival in Scotland 1971-1995*) found that, in comparison to other European countries, 'survival appears to have been worse in Scotland for cancers in which early diagnosis is the main influencing factor, and there is indirect evidence that patients in Scotland, at least in the past, tended to present with more advanced disease than their European counterparts.'[153]

*Evidence for all cancers*

Over 25,000 new cases of cancer were diagnosed in Scotland in 1998. Over the most recent ten-year period, incidence in men rose by 6.7 per cent and in women by 11.7 per cent. The corresponding figure was almost 117,000 in England. Table 5.3.1 presents incidence rates in England (alone) and Scotland for all malignant neoplasms, and for breast, lung, prostate, and colorectal cancers; the four major killers that account for more than half of all new cases.[154]

*Table 5.3.1*
**Cancer incidence by site in England and Scotland in 1998 (crude rates)**

| Cancer Site | England | | Scotland | | UK Rank | |
|---|---|---|---|---|---|---|
| | m | f | m | f | m | f |
| All cancers | 106,745 | 109,957 | 12,130 | 13,021 | N/A | N/A |
| Breast | 269 | 32,908 | 15 | 3,523 | 23 | 1 |
| Lung | 19,510 | 11,817 | 2,684 | 1,919 | 1 | 3 |
| Prostate | 19,335 | N/A | 1,795 | N/A | 2 | N/A |
| Colorectal | 15,173 | 13,848 | 1,835 | 1,589 | 3 | 2 |

*Source*: Cancer Research UK, Cancer statistics.

Table 5.3.2 shows age-standardised cancer incidence and mortality rates by year of diagnosis. As we saw in Tables 5.0.2A-D, mortality for both sexes is lower in England than in Scotland. Table 5.3.3 below shows some of the most recent cancer mortality statistics for England and Scotland (not including Wales). Note that deaths for men are higher than those for women for all cancers and also for major killers colorectal and lung cancer.

## Table 5.3.2
### Age-standardised (a) all cancer (ICD C00-C97), incidence and mortality rates by year of diagnosis

| | 1980 | 1985 | 1990 | 1991 | 1992 | 1993 | 1994 | 1995 | 1996 | 1997 | 1998 | 1999 |
|---|---|---|---|---|---|---|---|---|---|---|---|---|
| **Scotland (Male)** | | | | | | | | | | | | |
| - Incidence | N/A | N/A | 535.8 | 538.4 | 561.5 | 576.6 | 586.2 | 586.5 | 623.5 | 601.2 | 589.5 | 556.6 |
| - Mortality | | | 302.4 | 299.0 | 304.4 | 309.2 | 296.9 | 297.9 | 292.7 | 282.7 | 277.2 | 275.3 |
| **England (Male)** | | | | | | | | | | | | |
| - Incidence | 409.4 | 444.7 | 446.9 | 452.6 | 468.4 | 460.4 | 470.6 | N/A | N/A | N/A | N/A | N/A |
| - Mortality | 277.0 | 282.7 | 274.1 | 272.5 | 270.7 | 261.5 | 256.6 | 251.7 | 247.6 | 239.2 | 211.5 | 232.8 |
| **Scotland (Female)** | | | | | | | | | | | | |
| - Incidence | N/A | N/A | 424.1 | 422.7 | 437.6 | 440.9 | 445.4 | 451.6 | 480.2 | 480.8 | 467.9 | 452.7 |
| - Mortality | | | 202.3 | 199.3 | 200.9 | 202.8 | 202.9 | 198.3 | 197.8 | 193.5 | 190.3 | 190.1 |
| **England (Female)** | | | | | | | | | | | | |
| - Incidence | 304.9 | 339.2 | 357.7 | 365.3 | 378.9 | 364.5 | 372.6 | N/A | N/A | N/A | N/A | N/A |
| - Mortality | 178.0 | 185.3 | 182.0 | 181.0 | 179.8 | 175.4 | 173.0 | 170.6 | 169.3 | 165.9 | 162.7 | 161.8 |

*Sources: Trends in Cancer Survival in Scotland 1971-1995; Cancer Registration Statistics Scotland 1986-1995; SHOW – ISD online;
England 'Cancer Trends 1950-1999' (Figures are for England and Wales).*

(a) EASR: age-standardised incidence rate per 100,000 European Standard Population

## Table 5.3.3
## Selected cancer deaths and deaths under 75, in 2001, England and Scotland

|                        |       | All ages |          | Under 75 |          |
|------------------------|-------|----------|----------|----------|----------|
| Cancer (ICD10 numbers) |       | England  | Scotland | England  | Scotland |
| All cancer             | Men   | 67,601   | 7,819    | 35,590   | 4,579    |
| (C00-D48)              | Women | 62,916   | 7,584    | 30,216   | 3,828    |
|                        | Total | 130,517  | 15,475   | 65,806   | 8,407    |
| Colorectal cancer      | Men   | 6,981    | 835      | 3,746    | 475      |
| (C18-C20)              | Women | 6,225    | 780      | 2,360    | 305      |
|                        | Total | 13,206   | 1,615    | 6,106    | 780      |
| Lung cancer            | Men   | 16,567   | 2,277    | 9,350    | 1,425    |
| (C33, C34)             | Women | 10,454   | 1,638    | 5,602    | 941      |
|                        | Total | 27,021   | 3,915    | 14,952   | 2,366    |
| Breast cancer          | Men   | 77       | 7        | 36       | 5        |
| (C50)                  | Women | 10,627   | 1,143    | 5,839    | 679      |
|                        | Total | 10,704   | 1,150    | 5,875    | 684      |

*Source*: British Heart Foundation www.heartstat.org.uk
Original sources: ONS England, 2002 and GRO Edinburgh.

## Table 5.3.4A
## All cancer relative survival (%) at 1 year

|          | Sex    | 1971-75 | 1976-80 | 1981-85 | 1986-90 | 1991-95 |
|----------|--------|---------|---------|---------|---------|---------|
| England  | Male   | 37.0    | 39.8    | 46.4    | 50.9    | N/A     |
| Scotland | Male   | 35.1    | 38.5    | 43.0    | 47.4    | 51.8    |
| England  | Female | 52.4    | 54.4    | 59.1    | 62.1    | N/A     |
| Scotland | Female | 51.8    | 53.1    | 55.9    | 58.9    | 61.7    |

## Table 5.3.4B
## All cancer relative survival (%) at 5 years

|          | Sex    | 1971-75 | 1976-80 | 1981-85 | 1986-90 | 1991-95 |
|----------|--------|---------|---------|---------|---------|---------|
| England  | Male   | 19.1    | 22.5    | 27.6    | 31.4    | N/A     |
| Scotland | Male   | 21.3    | 23.3    | 26.0    | 29.9    | 33.9    |
| England  | Female | 31.7    | 35.2    | 39.7    | 43.4    | N/A     |
| Scotland | Female | 34.4    | 35.2    | 37.9    | 41.1    | 45.2    |

*Sources*: Scotland 'Trends in Cancer Survival in Scotland' (World Standard Population).
England: Coleman, M., Babb, P. *et al.*, *Cancer survival trends in England and Wales, 1971-1995*.[155] (England and Wales age-standardised population)

One- and five-year survival rates are shown in Tables 5.3.4A and B. While cancer incidence, deaths and survival rates are easily isolated for Scotland, it has been difficult to find published survival data for England that excludes Wales. Caution should be taken in interpreting survival data as the population standardisation differs between Scotland and England (and Wales), nevertheless trends may be observed with greater confidence. We can see that female survival is higher than that for males,[156] and that survival for all cancers (not only the major killers),[157] is slightly better in England. We also see that survival in England and Scotland has improved steadily since 1971-75. These improvements are not peculiar to the UK.

The tables in subsequent pages follow a regular order for each cancer site (lung, breast, colon/rectum, prostate, cervix, testis). Firstly, there is a snapshot of latest key statistics.[158] Secondly, we show incidence and mortality rates by year, age-standardised using the European Standard Population. English data are from Quinn, Babb *et al.*,[159] and include Wales. Scottish data are from ISD online (cancer facts and figures)[160] and *Cancer incidence and mortality by site/type of cancer, sex and year of diagnosis/registration of death: 1990-1999*, (formerly presented as part of *Scottish Health Statistics 2000*).

Finally, one- and five-year survival rates over time are shown. Scottish data are from *Trends in Cancer Survival in Scotland 1971-1995* and are standardised using the World Standard Population. Meanwhile, English figures are for England and Wales, and are taken from Quinn, Babb *et al.*,[161] and Coleman and Babb.[162] Readers will note that rates for one indicator (e.g. one-year survival) may differ from the same indicator in a different table for the same cancer site. This is caused by a number of factors, including the updating of data in sources published later, differing age-standardised populations, and the unavoidable inclusion in some cases of data from Wales. Therefore due caution should be taken when interpreting data.

## Lung cancer

Lung cancer is the most common cancer in men, the second most common in Scottish women, and the third most common in English women. It is the biggest cancer killer in the UK.[163] In 1999, lung cancer accounted for 26 per cent of cancer deaths in men and 17 per cent in women.[164] Tables 5.3.5, 5.3.6 and 5.3.7 show lung cancer data for England and Scotland. Incidence of lung cancer is decreasing in males and (more recently) females in England; indeed recently achieved decreases are reported be the fastest in the world.[165] However, in Scotland, although lung cancer incidence is falling among males it has been increasing among females—though it may have reached a plateau in 2000. These trends are expected to continue over the next decade.[166]

### Table 5.3.5
### Key statistics for lung cancer (ICD9, 162/ICD10 C33-34) incidence mortality and survival by sex and country, latest available year

| Indicator | Male | | Female | |
| --- | --- | --- | --- | --- |
| | Scotland | England | Scotland | England |
| Incidence | | | | |
| Number of cases | 2,835 | 19,600 | 2,023 | 11,500 |
| Incidence rate per 100,000 | | | | |
| Crude rate | 114.0 | 80.8 | 76.6 | 46.1 |
| ESR | 107.0 | 71.6 | 56.1 | 33.6 |
| WSR | 70.7 | 57.6 | 38.1 | 22.8 |
| Mortality | | | | |
| Number of deaths | 2,332 | 17,200 | 1,652 | 10,400 |
| Mortality rate per 100,000 | | | | |
| Crude rate | 93.9 | 70.4 | 62.7 | 41.6 |
| ESR | 85.8 | 61.3 | 43.7 | 28.9 |
| WSR | 56.0 | 39.5 | 29.1 | 19.2 |
| Relative survival (%) patients diagnosed in 1986-90 | | | | |
| One year | 19 | 21 | 19 | 20 |
| Five year | 6 | 6 | 6 | 6 |

*Source*: Quinn, M., Babb, P., Brock, A., Kirby, L., Jones, J, *Cancer Trends in England and Wales 1950-1999*, SMPS No. 66, London: ONS, 2001.
*Notes*: Scotland 1996 incidence, 1998 mortality; England, 1997 incidence, 1999 mortality. Figures for England are provisional. Incidence: 1995-1997, mortality: 1999.

In Scotland, incidence at all ages is amongst the highest in Europe and survival amongst the poorest.[167] Researchers have found that incidence and mortality rates for Scottish women have been the highest in Western Europe since 1950.[168] Differences in survival between the Scottish Health Boards are statistically significant; Greater Glasgow Health Board area has the highest incidence and mortality from lung cancer.[169] Similar patterns of geographic variation are also seen in England.

The most important risk factor for lung cancer is smoking. It is estimated that smoking causes around 90 per cent of cases.[170] If we look at tobacco consumption we see that smoking is more prevalent in Scotland (see Tables 2.4-2.6), though it has been declining in both men and women.

Lung cancer survival rates vary considerably in Europe. The lowest rates were again found in Denmark, Scotland and England, while the highest rates were found in France, the Netherlands and Switzerland. The EUROCARE II study showed that five-year survival rates for England and Wales were similar to those in Scotland; both are very poor. Lung cancer patients have seen small improvements in one-year survival, but survival five years post diagnosis has remained fairly stable over the past decade.

### Breast Cancer

Breast cancer is the most common female cancer in Scotland and England. The data in Tables 5.3.8 and 5.3.9 show little difference between breast cancer statistics in Scotland and England; mortality trends in Scotland have been similar to those in the rest of the UK since 1950,[171] though rates in Scotland are slightly higher.

Breast cancer mortality in the late 1980s in Scotland and England was among the highest in the world, though incidence was similar to other western countries.[172] Incidence rates in both counties are higher in least deprived populations. Mortality began to fall in the period after screening was introduced; that fall being larger in the 55-69 age-group.[173]

## Table 5.3.6

### Age-standardised (a) cancer of the trachea, bronchus and lung (ICD-10 C33-C34) incidence and mortality rates, per 100,000, by sex, age and year of diagnosis

|  | 1980 | 1985 | 1990 | 1991 | 1992 | 1993 | 1994 | 1995 | 1996 | 1997 | 1998 | 1999 | 2000 |
|---|---|---|---|---|---|---|---|---|---|---|---|---|---|
| **Scotland (Male)** | | | | | | | | | | | | | |
| Incidence | 135.3 | 132.5 | 116.6 | 117.8 | 119.8 | 117.2 | 112.9 | 108.5 | 108.1 | 102.7 | 101.1 | - | - |
| Mortality | - | - | - | 104.4 | 106.3 | 105.7 | 101.2 | 97.5 | 91.9 | 90.6 | 85.8 | 83.8 | 80.2 |
| **Scotland (Female)** | | | | | | | | | | | | | |
| Incidence | 35.8 | 45.0 | 49.4 | 49.0 | 52.5 | 50.2 | 50.9 | 51.9 | 56.5 | 53.7 | 54.4 | - | - |
| Mortality | - | - | - | 42.1 | 43.3 | 42.9 | 44.1 | 44.4 | 45.9 | 44.5 | 43.7 | 43.9 | 45.3 |
| **England (Male)** | | | | | | | | | | | | | |
| Incidence | 109.7 | 107.5 | 91.5 | 90.1 | 89.7 | 83.7 | 82.6 | 78.1 | 77.1 | 72.0 | - | - | |
| Mortality | 104.2 | 96.4 | 84.4 | 82.2 | 79.1 | 76.6 | 74.3 | 71.2 | 68.3 | 64.8 | 64.0 | 61.3 | |
| **England (Female)** | | | | | | | | | | | | | |
| Incidence | 27.1 | 32.0 | 32.7 | 32.8 | 33.9 | 33.2 | 33.7 | 34.4 | 35.6 | 33.7 | - | 28.8 | |
| Mortality | 25.0 | 27.4 | 28.9 | 29.3 | 29.1 | 29.4 | 29.6 | 29.6 | 29.4 | 28.5 | 29.1 | - | |

*Sources*: England 'Cancer Trends 1950-1999' (Figures are for England *and* Wales). Scotland, *Trends in Cancer Survival in Scotland 1971-1995*; Cancer Registration Statistics Scotland 1986-1995; SHOW – ISD online;

(a) Age-standardised incidence rate per 100,000, European standard population.

## Table 5.3.7
## Lung cancer survival (ICD162)

Relative survival (%) at one year

| Lung | Sex | 1971-75 | 1976-80 | 1981-85 | 1986-90 | 1991-95 en92-94 |
|---|---|---|---|---|---|---|
| England | Male | 15.0 | 15.0 | 18.0 | 19.0 | 20.6 |
| Scotland | Male | 16.4 | 16.4 | 18.5 | 19.9 | 21.4 |
| England | Female | 13.0 | 14.0 | 17.0 | 19.0 | 20.9 |
| Scotland | Female | 14.0 | 14.5 | 17.3 | 19.2 | 21.0 |

Relative survival (%) at five years

| Lung | Sex | 1971-75 | 1976-80 | 1981-85 | 1986-90 | 1991-95 |
|---|---|---|---|---|---|---|
| England | Male | 4.0 | 5.0 | 5.0 | 5.0 | 5.1 |
| Scotland | Male | 6.2 | 5.6 | 5.6 | 6.0 | 7.0 |
| England | Female | 4.0 | 4.0 | 5.0 | 5.0 | 5.3 |
| Scotland | Female | 5.5 | 4.9 | 5.6 | 6.2 | 6.4 |

*Sources*: Scotland 'Trends in Cancer Survival in Scotland' (World Standard Pop). England: Coleman, M., Babb, P. *et al.*, *Cancer survival trends in England and Wales, 1971-1995: deprivation and NHS Region*, ONS, Studies in Medical and Population Subjects No. 61, London: TSO, 1999. en92-94 figures are for England *only* and are taken from ONS Cancer Survival 1992-1999.

## Table 5.3.8
## Key statistics for female breast (ICD9 174, 175/ ICD10 C50) cancer incidence, mortality and survival by sex and country, latest available year

| Indicator | Scotland | England |
|---|---|---|
| Incidence | | |
| Number of cases | 3,242 | 30,800 |
| Incidence rate per 100,000 | | |
| Crude rate | 122.7 | 123.0 |
| ESR | 106.9 | 105.9 |
| WSR | 78.0 | 77.3 |
| Mortality | | |
| Number of deaths | 1,142 | 10,800 |
| Mortality rate per 100,000 | | |
| Crude rate | 43.3 | 43.0 |
| ESR | 33.0 | 31.8 |
| WSR | 22.9 | 22.0 |
| Relative survival (%) patients diagnosed in 1986-90 | | |
| One year | 90 | 90 |
| Five year | 67 | 68 |

*Source*: Quinn, M., Babb, P., Brock, A., Kirby, L. and Jones, J., *Cancer Trends in England and Wales 1950-1999*, SMPS, No. 66, London: ONS, 2001.
*Notes*: Scotland 1996 incidence, 1998 mortality; England 1997 incidence, 1999 mortality. Figures for England are provisional. Incidence: 1995-1997, mortality: 1999.

## Table 5.3.9
### *Age-standardised breast cancer (ICD-10 C50) mortality and incidence rates, per 100,000 women by year of diagnosis*

| | 1980 | 1985 | 1990 | 1991 | 1992 | 1993 | 1994 | 1995 | 1996 | 1997 | 1998 | 1999 | 2000 |
|---|---|---|---|---|---|---|---|---|---|---|---|---|---|
| **Scotland** | | | | | | | | | | | | | |
| Incidence | 83.7 | 84.4 | 100.4 | 108.2 | 110.3 | 105.2 | 104.1 | 109.4 | 108.5 | 112.7 | 115.7 | N/A | N/A |
| Mortality | 39.8 | 38.9 | 37.4 | 38.2 | 37.9 | 38.0 | 38.3 | 36.4 | 34.2 | 33.6 | 33.0 | 32.3 | 31.4 |
| **England** | | | | | | | | | | | | | |
| Incidence | 77.8 | 85.7 | 98.4 | 105.1 | 107.6 | 101.4 | 104.7 | 101.8 | 104.0 | 107.0 | N/A | N/A | N/A |
| Mortality | 39.3 | 40.2 | 39.0 | 38.6 | 38.0 | 37.5 | 36.8 | 35.7 | 34.4 | 33.5 | 32.6 | NA | N/A |

*Sources:* Scotland, *Trends in Cancer Survival in Scotland 1971-1995;* Cancer Registration Statistics Scotland 1986-1995; SHOW – ISD online; England 'Cancer Trends 1950-1999' (Figures are for England and Wales).
Mortality figures based on EASR: age-standardised incidence rate per 100,000 European Standard Population

Table 5.3.10 shows that one- and five-year breast cancer survival rates are similar in England and Scotland; improvements over time are reflected in declining mortality. Four groups emerged when breast cancer survival was compared in the EUROCARE II Study. Switzerland and France were in the best performing group, Denmark, the Netherlands and Germany in the second group. Scotland and England (with Slovenia) were below average in a third group, while Slovakia, Poland and Estonia were in the worst performing group. While most countries presented a stable or increasing survival rate with increasing age of patients, England, Scotland, Slovakia, Poland and Estonia showed lower survival for the elderly,[174] perhaps suggesting age-based rationing. Of eight countries (not including Scotland) for which data were collected by the OECD in 2002, England had the lowest five-year survival rate overall. And for patients aged 80 or more there was a huge gap in the survival rate (53 per cent compared with the next worst country, Canada with 68 per cent).[175] This again suggests that older women in England are being written off because 'they've had a good innings'.[176]

Since the publication of the EUROCARE II study, deaths from breast cancer have fallen in the UK. Since 1990, the death rate from breast cancer has fallen by about 30 per cent overall.[177] Accordingly, five-year survival rates have seen significant improvements. It is suggested that much of the improvement in Britain's performance can be accounted for by the use of adjuvant treatments after surgery—tamoxifen, chemotherapy, and well-targeted radiotherapy.[178] 'Tamoxifen may particularly help to explain Britain's lead because British doctors adopted its widespread use in around 1985, earlier than in the US or other European countries.'[179] In Scotland, the use of adjuvant systemic therapy increased from 70 per cent of patients treated surgically to 96 per cent between 1987 and 1993.[180]

## Colorectal Cancer

Colorectal cancer (ICD 9 153+154; ICD-10 C18-20) is the third most common cancer in England and in Scotland for both sexes. It is the second most common cause of cancer death for both sexes. Incidence of, mortality and survival from colorectal cancer are shown in Tables 5.3.11-5.3.13. Roughly two-thirds of these cancers are of the colon, the remainder are of the rectum.

**Table 5.3.10**
**Age-standardised breast cancer survival**
**ICD9 174/ICD-10 C50**

Relative survival (%) at one year

| Breast | Sex | 1971-75 | 1976-80 | 1981-85 | 1986-90 | 1991-95(a) |
|---|---|---|---|---|---|---|
| England | Female | 82.0 | 85.0 | 87.0 | 89.0 | 92.3 |
| Scotland | Female | 84.3 | 87.3 | 87.5 | 89.6 | 91.2 |

Relative survival (%) at five years

| Breast | Sex | 1971-75 | 1976-80 | 1981-85 | 1986-90 | 1991-95 |
|---|---|---|---|---|---|---|
| England | Female | 52.0 | 54.0 | 58.0 | 66.0 | 75.0 |
| Scotland | Female | 56.8 | 60.4 | 62.8 | 66.0 | 72.8 |

*Sources*: Scotland 'Trends in Cancer Survival in Scotland' (World Standard Pop). England: Coleman, Babb, *et al.*, *Cancer survival trends in England and Wales, 1971-1995: deprivation and NHS Region*, 1999. (a) Figures for England are for 1992-1994 *only* and are taken from ONS Cancer Survival 1992-1999.

Incidence in Scotland has risen significantly for males and is higher than England (and Sweden, Spain, the Netherlands, Italy, Germany, France, Finland, Denmark and the USA). These trends may reflect the Scottish male diet—as colorectal cancer is mainly associated with developed countries and diets low in fruit, vegetables and fibre and high in fats and animal proteins (see Table 2.7). Overall, males in England and females in both England and Scotland have seen small rises in incidence followed by modest falls. Mortality rates have fallen over the past 20 years, but mortality is again higher among Scottish males and has remained fairly level since 1985.

*Table 5.3.11*
**Key statistics for colorectal (ICD9 153-154/ICD-10 C18-21)
cancer incidence, mortality and survival by sex and country,
latest available year**

|  | Male | | Female | |
| Indicator | Scotland | England | Scotland | England |
| --- | --- | --- | --- | --- |
| Incidence | | | | |
| Number of cases | 1,846 | 13,900 | 1,765 | 13,000 |
| Incidence rate per 100,000 | | | | |
| Crude rate | 74.3 | 57.3 | 66.8 | 52.1 |
| ESR | 70.3 | 51.2 | 45.9 | 34.6 |
| WSR | 46.2 | 33.8 | 30.4 | 22.8 |
| Mortality | | | | |
| Number of deaths | 857 | 6,940 | 803 | 6,630 |
| Mortality rate per 100,000 | | | | |
| Crude rate | 34.5 | 28.5 | 30.5 | 26.4 |
| ESR | 31.9 | 24.9 | 19.2 | 16.1 |
| WSR | 20.5 | 15.9 | 12.3 | 10.3 |
| Relative survival (%) patients diagnosed in 1986-90 | | | | |
| One year | 61 | 61 | 59 | 60 |
| Five year | 40 | 39 | 40 | 39 |

*Source*: Quinn, Babb, Brock, Kirby and Jones, *Cancer Trends in England and Wales 1950-1999*, 2001.

*Notes*: Scotland 1996 incidence, 1998 mortality; England, 1997 Incidence, 1999 mortality. Figures for England are provisional. Incidence: 1995-1997, mortality: 1999.

For colorectal cancer, survival rates collected by EURO-CARE II were high in the Netherlands, Switzerland and France, while Eastern European countries, Scotland, England and Denmark had low survival rates.[181] The US compares favourably with the best European countries for cancer survival.[182] One- and five-year survival have increased significantly in England and Scotland over the past 25 years. However, despite these improvements survival is still significantly worse than the estimated European average.[183] Survival is also worse for those patients from most deprived groups in both England and Scotland.[184]

## Table 5.3.12
### *Age-standardised (a) colorectal cancer, incidence and mortality rates, per 100,000, by sex and year of diagnosis*

| | 1980 | 1985 | 1990 | 1991 | 1992 | 1993 | 1994 | 1995 | 1996 | 1997 | 1998 | 1999 | 2000 |
|---|---|---|---|---|---|---|---|---|---|---|---|---|---|
| **Scotland (Male)** | | (b) | | | | | | | | | | | |
| Incidence | N/A | 55.9 | 57.3 | 60.3 | 61.2 | 63.2 | 63.0 | 62.0 | 70.2 | 68.1 | 67.1 | N/A | N/A |
| Mortality | | 30.3 | 32.0 | 33.1 | 33.9 | 34.5 | 33.8 | 31.0 | 32.8 | 33.3 | 31.5 | 32.2 | 30.4 |
| **Scotland (Female)** | | | | | | | | | | | | | |
| Incidence | N/A | 41.5 | 43.1 | 39.7 | 39.2 | 43.1 | 43.2 | 43.0 | 45.2 | 40.9 | 40.7 | N/A | N/A |
| Mortality | | 23.4 | 22.7 | 23.1 | 21.5 | 22.7 | 21.3 | 21.7 | 20.7 | 18.5 | 18.9 | 18.9 | 17.5 |
| **England (Male)** | | | | | | | | | | | | | |
| Incidence | 47.2 | 50.7 | 51.9 | 51.6 | 54.6 | 53.9 | 53.0 | 50.6 | 53.2 | 51.6 | N/A | N/A | N/A |
| Mortality | 30.4 | 30.1 | 29.6 | 29.1 | 29.6 | 29.3 | 28.2 | 27.9 | 27.3 | 26.7 | 26.2 | 25.1 | N/A |
| **England (Female)** | | | | | | | | | | | | | |
| Incidence | 34.8 | 36.3 | 35.5 | 35.6 | 37.4 | 35.5 | 35.6 | 33.7 | 36.4 | 34.8 | N/A | N/A | N/A |
| Mortality | 23.2 | 21.9 | 19.6 | 19.4 | 19.3 | 19.0 | 18.6 | 17.8 | 17.5 | 16.9 | 16.2 | 16.1 | N/A |

*Sources: Trends in Cancer Survival in Scotland 1971-1995; Cancer Registration Statistics Scotland 1986-1995, SHOW – ISD online; England 'Cancer Trends 1950-1999' (Figures are for England and Wales).*

*Notes:* (a) ASR: age-standardised incidence rate per 100,000 European Standard Population; (b) Scottish figures for 1989.

### Table 5.3.13
### Colon cancer survival (ICD 153)

Relative survival (%) at one year

| Colon Cancer | Sex | 1971-75 | 1976-80 | 1981-85 | 1986-90 | 1991-95 |
|---|---|---|---|---|---|---|
| England | Male | 39.0 | 45.0 | 54.0 | 59.0 | N/A |
| Scotland | Male | 41.1 | 48.6 | 52.6 | 59.8 | 64.0 |
| England | Female | 40.0 | 45.0 | 54.0 | 59.0 | N/A |
| Scotland | Female | 41.4 | 44.2 | 52.5 | 57.7 | 63.4 |

Relative survival (%) at five years

| Colorectal Cancer | Sex | 1971-75 | 1976-80 | 1981-85 | 1986-90 | 1991-95 |
|---|---|---|---|---|---|---|
| England | Male | 22.0 | 28.0 | 35.0 | 38.0 | N/A |
| Scotland | Male | 26.8 | 31.7 | 34.2 | 39.8 | 44.6 |
| England | Female | 23.0 | 28.0 | 35.0 | 39.0 | N/A |
| Scotland | Female | 26.7 | 28.7 | 34.2 | 39.7 | 44.9 |

Sources: Scotland 'Trends in Cancer Survival in Scotland' (World Standard Pop). England: Coleman, Babb, et al., Cancer survival trends in England and Wales, 1971-1995: deprivation and NHS Region, 1999.

## Prostate Cancer

Prostate cancer is the second most common cancer in the Scots and the English and its incidence is increasing in the UK.[185] Incidence is higher among Scots, though mortality is similar, and has risen slightly over the past 20 years in both countries (see Tables 5.3.14 - 5.3.16). Scottish incidence is in a middle range of certain comparator countries (Sweden, Spain, the Netherlands, Italy, Germany, France, Finland, Denmark and the USA).

Table 5.3.14 shows Scottish one- and five-year survival is better than that in England; five-year relative survival in England and Wales in the late 1980s was six percentage points lower than Scotland.[186] Table 5.3.16 shows improving survival rates over time. However, on an international level, we should remember that the EUROCARE II study found that the lowest survival rates for prostate cancer were seen in the Eastern European countries, the UK and Denmark, while the highest survival rates were again found in Switzerland.[187] Survival rates are lower in both England and Scotland for the most deprived.[188]

*Table 5.3.14*
## *Key statistics for prostate cancer (ICD9 185/ICD10 C61) incidence, mortality and survival by sex and country, latest available year*

| Indicator | Scotland | England |
|---|---|---|
| Incidence | | |
|     Number of cases | 2,030 | 17,200 |
| Incidence rate per 100,000 | | |
|     Crude rate | 81.7 | 70.7 |
|     ESR | 75.3 | 60.7 |
|     WSR | 46.9 | 32.9 |
| Mortality | | |
|     Number of deaths | 667 | 8,020 |
| Mortality rate per 100,000 | | |
|     Crude rate | 27.3 | 32.9 |
|     ESR | 25.1 | 27.3 |
|     WSR | 14.6 | 15.7 |
| Relative survival (%) patients diagnosed in 1986-90 | | |
|     One year | 81 | 78 |
|     Five year | 49 | 42 |

*Source:* Quinn, Babb, Brock, Kirby and Jones, *Cancer Trends in England and Wales 1950-1999*, 2001.

*Notes:* Scotland 1996 incidence, 1998 mortality; England, 1997 incidence, 1999 mortality. Figures for England are provisional: incidence: 1995-1997, mortality, 1999.

## Table 5.3.15

### Age-standardised (a) prostate cancer, incidence and mortality rates per 100,000, by year of diagnosis

| | 1980 | 1985 | 1989 | 1990 | 1991 | 1992 | 1993 | 1994 | 1995 | 1996 | 1997 | 1998 | 1999 | 2000 |
|---|---|---|---|---|---|---|---|---|---|---|---|---|---|---|
| **Scotland** | | | | | | | | | | | | | | |
| Incidence | N/A | N/A | 49.7 | 52.4 | 51.9 | 55.4 | 66.6 | 68.7 | 71.5 | 77.9 | 70.1 | 67.2 | N/A | N/A |
| Mortality | N/A | N/A | N/A | N/A | 25.4 | 26.7 | 29.2 | 28.8 | 29.2 | 28.0 | 26.1 | 25.1 | 28.0 | 27.6 |
| **England** | | | | | | | | | | | | | | |
| Incidence | 36.5 | 42.4 | 46.0 | 47.4 | 49.8 | 54.5 | 58.9 | 66.1 | 63.2 | 64.4 | 60.7 | N/A | N/A | N/A |
| Mortality | 21.1 | 24.2 | 26.8 | 27.0 | 28.2 | 28.3 | 29.5 | 29.3 | 29.5 | 28.8 | 27.6 | 27.4 | 27.3 | N/A |

Sources: *Trends in Cancer Survival in Scotland 1971-1995*; Cancer Registration Statistics Scotland 1986-1995; SHOW – ISD online; England 'Cancer Trends 1950-1999' (Figures are for England and Wales).
(a) EASR: age-standardised incidence rate per 100,000 European Standard Population

## Table 5.3.16

### Prostate cancer survival (ICD 185)

| Relative survival (%) at one year | 1971-75 | 1976-80 | 1981-85 | 1986-90 | 1991-95(a) |
|---|---|---|---|---|---|
| **Prostate** | | | | | |
| England | 65.0 | 69.0 | 76.0 | 76.0 | 81.0 |
| Scotland | 63.8 | 66.2 | 70.5 | 73.4 | 75.7 |

| Relative survival (%) at five years | 1971-75 | 1976-80 | 1981-85 | 1986-90 | 1991-95 |
|---|---|---|---|---|---|
| **Prostate** | | | | | |
| England | 31.0 | 37.0 | 41.0 | 41.0 | 54.9 |
| Scotland | 36.7 | 38.4 | 39.5 | 42.5 | 49.6 |

Sources: Scotland 'Trends in Cancer Survival in Scotland' (World Standard Pop). England: Coleman, Babb, *et al.*, *Cancer survival trends in England and Wales, 1971-1995: deprivation and NHS Region*, 1999.
(a) Figures for England are for 1992-1994 only and are taken from ONS Cancer Survival 1992-1999.

## Cervical Cancer

The incidence of cervical cancer is closely related to sexual behaviour. Quinn, Babb *et al.* note that: 'Very low rates of the disease occur in nuns'.[189] It is the most common cancer in women aged 25-29. There have been steady declines in both incidence and mortality since 1990 in both countries. Mortality rates in Scotland are similar to those in England, though incidence rates have not fallen as far as English rates (see Tables 5.3.17-5.3.19).

*Table 5.3.17*
*Key statistics for cervical cancer (ICD 9/ICD10 C53)*
*incidence, mortality and survival by sex and country,*
*latest available year*

| Indicator | | Scotland | England |
|---|---|---|---|
| Incidence | Number of cases | 341 | 2,670 |
| Incidence rate per 100,000 | | | |
| | Crude rate | 14.4 | 10.7 |
| | ESR | 12.9 | 9.6 |
| | WSR | 10.3 | 7.7 |
| Mortality | | | |
| | Number of deaths | 145 | 1,030 |
| Mortality rate per 100,000 | | | |
| | Crude rate | 5.5 | 4.1 |
| | ESR | 4.2 | 3.3 |
| | WSR | 3.0 | 2.4 |
| Relative survival (%) patients diagnosed in 1986-90 | | | |
| | One year | 83 | 83 |
| | Five year | 63 | 64 |

*Source*: Quinn, Babb, Brock, Kirby and Jones, *Cancer Trends in England and Wales 1950-1999*, 2001.
*Notes*: Scotland 1996 incidence, 1998 mortality; England, 1997 Incidence, 1999 mortality. Figures for England are provisional. Incidence: 1995-1997, mortality: 1999.

In contrast to other cancers, both Scottish and English cervical cancer incidence, mortality and survival fall in a middle range of certain comparator countries (Sweden, Spain, the Netherlands, Italy, Germany, France, Finland, Denmark and the USA).[190]

Survival rates shown in Table 5.3.17 show little difference between England and Scotland (diagnosis between 1986-1990), while those in Table 5.3.19 suggest survival is rather better in England. These figures should be treated with caution, as the age-standardisation population used in our sources was different. Nevertheless, improvement trends can be observed.

The EUROCARE II study found five-year survival for gynaecological tumours (cervical and ovarian cancer) generally to be higher in the Netherlands and Switzerland than in other European countries.[191] Researchers concluded that differences in survival for cervical cancer are almost certainly related to differences between screening programmes—given that screening can aid diagnosis of asymptomatic malignant disease, and that early diagnosis allows early treatment.[192] Further details of Scottish and English screening programmes are given below.

There is strong evidence in Scotland of trends of higher incidence and mortality rates and lower survival of those patients of lower socio-economic status.[193]

124

## Table 5.3.18
### Age-standardised (a) cervical cancer (ICDC53), incidence and mortality rates per 100,000 by sex and year of diagnosis

| | 1980 | 1985 | 1989 | 1990 | 1991 | 1992 | 1993 | 1994 | 1995 | 1996 | 1997 | 1998 | 1999 | 2000 |
|---|---|---|---|---|---|---|---|---|---|---|---|---|---|---|
| **Scotland** | | | | | | | | | | | | | | |
| Incidence | 14.5 | 16.3 | 13.5 | 18.0 | 16.8 | 14.1 | 13.7 | 12.4 | 12.0 | 13.0 | 12.6 | 12.8 | N/A | N/A |
| Mortality | N/A | N/A | N/A | N/A | 5.9 | 5.9 | 5.4 | 4.9 | 4.6 | 4.2 | 4.4 | 4.2 | 3.8 | 3.5 |
| **England** | | | | | | | | | | | | | | |
| Incidence | 15.3 | 16.4 | 15.7 | 15.4 | 12.8 | 12.0 | 11.6 | 11.0 | 10.3 | 9.7 | 9.6 | N/A | N/A | N/A |
| Mortality | 6.9 | 6.3 | 5.1 | 5.5 | 5.2 | 5.0 | 4.7 | 4.2 | 4.1 | 4.1 | 3.7 | 3.5 | 3.3 | N/A |

Sources: Trends in Cancer Survival in Scotland 1971-1995; Cancer Registration Statistics Scotland 1986-1995; SHOW – ISD online;
England 'Cancer Trends 1950-1999' (Figures are for England and Wales).
(a) EASR: age-standardised incidence rate per 100,000 European Standard Population

## Table 5.3.19
### Cervical cancer survival rates in Scotland and England, (ICD 180 – cervix uteri)

Relative survival rate (%) at one year

| Cervical and Ovarian | 1971-75 | 1976-80 | 1981-85 | 1986-90 | 1991-95 en92-94 |
|---|---|---|---|---|---|
| England | 75.0 | 76.0 | 80.0 | 82.0 | 83.7 |
| Scotland | 75.3 | 74.1 | 75.2 | 73.4 | 75.7 |

Relative survival (%) at five years

| Cervical and Ovarian | 1971-75 | 1976-80 | 1981-85 | 1986-90 | 1991-95 |
|---|---|---|---|---|---|
| England | 52.0 | 54.0 | 58.0 | 58.0 | 65.2 |
| Scotland | 36.7 | 38.4 | 39.5 | 42.5 | 49.6 |

*Sources*: Scotland 'Trends in Cancer Survival in Scotland' (World Standard Pop). England: Coleman, Babb *et al.*, *Cancer survival trends in England and Wales, 1971-1995: deprivation and NHS* 1999. en92-94 figures are for England only and are taken from ONS Cancer Survival 1992-1999.

## Testicular Cancer

Incidence of cancer of the testis is slightly higher in Scotland than England and has risen marginally over the past 20 years. In December 2002, the BBC reported that, overall, cancer mortality in the UK had fallen every year between 1983 and 2000. The most dramatic success was for testicular cancer: mortality fell by 15 per cent in five years, even though the number of cases had risen. Tables 5.3.20 and 5.3.21 set out some key statistics for testicular cancer.

Survival for patients with testicular cancer is good in Scotland and England and all our comparator countries (Sweden, Spain, the Netherlands, Italy, Germany, France, Finland, Denmark and the USA) for which we have data. One- and five-year survival in Scotland is almost identical to that in England. Survival rose significantly in the 1970s as new treatments were introduced (see Table 5.3.22).[194]

## Geographical Variation in Cancer Incidence and Survival

Geographical variation in cancer incidence and mortality rates and survival is significant in both England and Scotland, as is variation by deprivation.[195] The Carstairs Deprivation Index reveals a mixed picture depending on which cancer is being examined. Those living in deprived areas may not survive as long as the more affluent. The strongest evidence of this is for lung cancer, but in 38 out of 43 cancers studied in England and Wales there is a 'gap in survival to the advantage of the most affluent'.[196] This pattern is a feature of cancer in both England and Scotland and thus tells us little about differences between the two. Further study of survival by deprivation in England, Scotland and other countries would be required if firm conclusions were to be made about the reasons for these gradients.

*Table 5.3.20*
*Key statistics for testicular cancer (ICD9 180/ICD10 C53)*
*incidence, mortality and survival by sex and country,*
*latest available year*

| Indicator | | Scotland | England |
|---|---|---|---|
| Incidence | | | |
| | Number of cases | 169 | 1,370 |
| Incidence rate per 100,000 | | | |
| | Crude rate | 6.8 | 5.6 |
| | ESR | 6.3 | 5.4 |
| | WSR | 5.9 | 4.6 |
| Mortality | | | |
| | Number of deaths | 11 | 70 |
| Mortality rate per 100,000 | | | |
| | Crude rate | 0.4 | 0.3 |
| | ESR | 0.4 | 0.3 |
| | WSR | 0.4 | 0.2 |
| Relative survival (%) patients diagnosed in 1996-90 | | | |
| | One year | 95 | 96 |
| | Five year | 92 | 91 |

*Source*: Quinn, Babb, Brock, Kirby and Jones, *Cancer Trends in England and Wales 1950-1999*, 2001.

*Notes*: Scotland 1996 incidence, 1998 mortality; England, 1997 incidence, 1999 mortality. Figures for England are provisional. Incidence: 1995-1997, mortality: 1999.

## Table 5.3.21
### Age-standardised (a) testicular cancer (ICDC62), incidence and mortality rates, per 100,000, by year of diagnosis

| | 1980 | 1985 | 1989 | 1990 | 1991 | 1992 | 1993 | 1994 | 1995 | 1996 | 1997 | 1998 | 1999 | 2000 |
|---|---|---|---|---|---|---|---|---|---|---|---|---|---|---|
| **Scotland** | | | | | | | | | | | | | | |
| Incidence | N/A | N/A | 6.0 | 6.4 | 6.6 | 6.1 | 6.2 | 7.5 | 6.3 | 6.3 | 7.1 | 8.0 | N/A | N/A |
| Mortality | 1.1 | 0.5 | 0.4 | 0.6 | 0.4 | 0.4 | 0.6 | 0.3 | 0.3 | 0.4 | 0.2 | 0.4 | 0.3 | 0.4 |
| **England** | | | | | | | | | | | | | | |
| Incidence | 3.7 | 4.3 | 5.1 | 4.8 | 5.2 | 5.3 | 5.3 | 5.2 | 5.6 | 5.7 | 5.4 | N/A | N/A | N/A |
| Mortality | 0.8 | 0.4 | 0.4 | 0.5 | 0.4 | 0.4 | 0.4 | 0.3 | 0.3 | 0.4 | 0.2 | 0.3 | 0.3 | N/A |

*Sources: Trends in Cancer Survival in Scotland 1971-1995*, Cancer Registration Statistics Scotland 1986-1995; SHOW – ISD online; England 'Cancer Trends 1950-1999' (Figures are for England and Wales).
(a) EASR: age-standardised incidence rate per 100,000 European standard population

**Table 5.3.22**
**Age-standardised (a) testicular cancer (ICDC62)**
**survival rates by year of diagnosis**

Relative survival (%) at one year

| Testicular | 1971-75 | 1976-80 | 1981-85 | 1986-90 | 1991-95 |
|---|---|---|---|---|---|
| England | 82.0 | 85.0 | 94.0 | 95.0 | N/A |
| Scotland | 81.1 | 86.2 | 94.3 | 95.3 | 96.3 |

Relative survival (%) at five years

| Testicular | 1971-75 | 1976-80 | 1981-85 | 1986-90 | 1991-95 |
|---|---|---|---|---|---|
| England | 69.0 | 78.0 | 88.0 | 90.0 | N/A |
| Scotland | 67.5 | 74.1 | 87.3 | 91.7 | 93.5 |

*Sources*: Scotland 'Trends in Cancer Survival in Scotland' (World Standard Pop). England: Coleman, Babb *et al.*, *Cancer survival trends in England and Wales, 1971-1995: deprivation and NHS Region*, 1999.
(a) Standardised to the age-group 15-74 rather than 15-99, because of small numbers in older age-groups

## *Summary*

Cancer outcomes in England and Scotland present something of a mixed picture. It is difficult to say that one country is better than the other at dealing with cancer, particularly as performance varies between cancers, and between sexes, not to mention between regions and between those of different socio-economic status. However, Tables 5.3.23 and 5.3.24 summarise our cancer evidence by ranking survival rates. Taking into account this rather limited collection of cancers, and bearing in mind that differences in survival rates between countries and sexes are very small indeed (usually c. one per cent), Table 5.3.23 shows that Scotland appears to perform fractionally better than England for some cancers (most notably for prostate cancer) and fractionally worse for others (including cervical cancer). Overall, for this group of cancers English men seem to fare slightly less well than Scots, while English women appear to have very slightly better survival rates than the Scots.

## Table 5.3.23
### Cancer survival rankings according to snapshot tables(combined picture of one- and five-year rates). Diagnosed 1986-90, survival rates in parenthesis

| Cancer | | Scotland | | England | |
|---|---|---|---|---|---|
| | | Male | Female | Male | Female |
| Lung | one year | 3 (19) | 3 (19) | 1(21) | 2(20) |
| | five year | 1 (6) | 1 (6) | 1 (6) | 1 (6) |
| Breast | one year | N/A | 1(90) | N/A | 1(90) |
| | five year | N/A | 2(67) | N/A | 1(68) |
| Colorectal | one year | 1(61) | 4(59) | 1(61) | 3(60) |
| | five year | 1(40) | 1(40) | 3(39) | 3(39) |
| Prostate | one year | 1(81) | N/A | 2(78) | N/A |
| | five year | 1(49) | N/A | 2(42) | N/A |
| Cervix | one year | N/A | 1(83) | N/A | 1(83) |
| | five year | N/A | 2(63) | N/A | 1(64) |
| Testis | one year | 2(95) | N/A | 1(96) | N/A |
| | five year | 1(92) | N/A | 2(91) | N/A |

*Source*: Civitas research findings. This comparison of cancer data indicates trends, but does not stand close scrutiny owing to concerns over comparability of data.

## Table 5.3.24
### Cancer survival rankings summary of remaining survival tables (combined picture of one-and five-year rates) (92-94 figures for England are not included)

| Cancer | | Scotland | | England | |
|---|---|---|---|---|---|
| | | Male | Female | Male | Female |
| All cancer | one year | 4 | 2 | 3 | 1 |
| | five year | 4 | 2 | 3 | 1 |
| Lung | one year | 1 | 2 | 2 | 2 |
| | five year | 1 | 1 | 3 | 3 |
| Breast | one year | N/A | 1 | N/A | 2 |
| | five year | N/A | 1 | N/A | 1 |
| Colorectal | one year | 1 | 4 | 2 | 2 |
| | five year | 1 | 1 | 4 | 3 |
| Prostate | one year | 2 | N/A | 1 | N/A |
| | five year | 1 | N/A | 2 | N/A |
| Cervix | one year | N/A | 2 | N/A | 1 |
| | five year | N/A | 2 | N/A | 1 |
| Testis | one year | 1 | N/A | 1 | N/A |
| | five year | 1 | N/A | 2 | N/A |

*Source*: Civitas research findings. This comparison of cancer data indicates trends, but does not stand close scrutiny owing to concerns over comparability of data.

Table 5.3.24, though requiring more cautious interpretation owing to the inconsistent age-standardisation of data, presents a similar picture of English women fairing slightly better than Scots women and English men fairing slightly worse than Scots men though slightly better if survival from 'all cancers' is considered. While we emphasise that the rankings set out above are imperfect, and there is perhaps no firm lesson to learn from comparing cancer outcomes in Scotland and England, we can put those outcomes in an international context with greater confidence. Table 5.3.25 summarises the above evidence by splitting a number of comparator countries into groups according to cancer survival. UK performance as a whole, along with that of Denmark, is weak.

**Table 5.3.25**
***Cancer care survival groups (all cancers)***

| Group one<br>Low survival rates | Group two | Group three | Group four<br>High survival rates |
|---|---|---|---|
| Eastern European<br>Countries | UK<br>England<br>Scotland<br>Denmark | Germany<br>Netherlands | USA<br>Switzerland<br>France |

Source: derived from ISD Scotland, *Trends in Cancer Survival Scotland: 1971-95*; Quinn, Babb *et al.*, *Cancer Trends 1950-99*; Eurocare II study results.

## Cancer Treatment

Survival rates among US cancer patients are higher when compared to those of European patients. These findings are particularly notable for breast cancer, but also other cancers for which treatment and screening can make a difference.[197] Cancer care resources may lie behind these figures; it has long been accepted that cancer care is under-resourced in the UK. Professor Karol Sikora, former head of the World Health Organisation's cancer programme, has summed up the situation in the UK as follows: 'We know that Britain has fewer radiotherapists per head than Poland and fewer medical oncologists than any country in Western Europe. ... Britain is a significantly lower user of chemotherapy than its neighbours. Rationing cancer drugs is commonplace.'[198] What differences can be observed between Scotland and England? The following section sets out some of the evidence on referral times, availability of diagnostic and treatment equipment, numbers of specialists, cancer screening, radiation therapy, and rates of surgical resection for lung cancer.

## Referral Times

One key to diagnosis and treatment outcome is referral time. The picture *vis á vis* referral times is improving in both Scotland and England. *The Annual Report (2003) of the NHS Modernisation Board* announces that in England: 'Between October 2001 and September 2002, some 96 per cent [323,000] of suspected cancer patients were seen by a specialist within two weeks of being urgently referred by their GP'; an increase from 91 per cent in the previous year.[199] Figures from March 2003 show that between October and December 2002 almost 98 per cent of GP referrals see a specialist within two weeks.[200]

In the year to December 2002, 94.4 per cent of breast cancer patients received their first treatment within one month of diagnosis. The NHS Plan target is 100 per cent by 2005. Treatment is received within one month of diagnosis by 99 per cent of leukaemia sufferers and 93.4 per cent of those with testicular cancer.[201]

Meanwhile, in Scotland *Action for Change* contains commitments on referral and subsequent treatment waiting times. For example: 'By October 2001, women who have breast cancer and are referred for urgent treatment will begin that treatment within one month of diagnosis, where clinically appropriate.'[202] There is a general target that by 2005 the maximum wait from urgent referral to treatment for all cancers will be two months.[203] And recognising the importance of rapid diagnosis, Scotland has at least 137 one-stop clinics providing rapid diagnosis facilities.[204] Treatment guidelines have been published for a number of cancers. The Scottish Cancer Group has also commissioned a number of reports on radiology, medical and clinical oncology, radiotherapy, and palliative care.

## Number of Specialist Cancer Staff

Cancer specialists may be surgeons, clinical oncologists (trained in both radiotherapy and chemotherapy), or medical oncologists (trained in chemotherapy only). Tables 5.3.26 and 5.3.27 show numbers and rates of medical and clinical oncologists (sometimes know as non-surgical oncologists) in Scotland and England. We see that Scotland has a slight advantage over England in the rates of clinical and medical oncologists per million. There is significant geographical variation in numbers per cancer unit.[205]

The Annual Report (2003) of the English NHS Modernisation Board states that: 'Figures for March 2002 show that 3,864 cancer consultants were in posts in March 2002 compared to 3,362 at September 1999—an increase of 502 (15 per cent)'. This rise is on target to meet the NHS Plan pledge to increase the number of cancer consultants by 1,000 by 2006.[206] However, despite some progress in recruitment, the 'the lack of trained staff remains the biggest single problem' and as a result the cancer workforce works under great pressure. The report continues: 'We particularly need more doctors, nurses, radiographers, biomedical scientists and administrative support staff.'[207] In March 2002 6.4 per cent of clinical oncology posts were vacant in England; in some regions vacancies were over ten per cent (Northern and Yorkshire, West Midlands, and North West).

### Table 5.3.26
### Medical and clinical oncologists numbers and whole time equivalents (per million population in parenthesis)

|  | 2000 (Number) | 200 ( WTE) | 2002 (Number) | 2002 (WTE) |
|---|---|---|---|---|
| Medical Oncology |  |  |  |  |
| England | 133 (2.7) | 103 (2.1) | N/A | N/A |
| Scotland | 14 (2.7) | 11.1 (2.2) | 16 (3.1) | 13.7 (2.7) |
| Clinical Oncology |  |  |  |  |
| England | 307 (6.2) | 279 (5.7) | 330 (6.7) (a) | N/A |
| Scotland | 38 (7.5) | 34.5 (6.7) | 39 (7.6) | 36.3 (7.1) |

Source: Medical and Dental Census ISD Scotland; DoH, Hospital, Public Health Medicine and Community Health Services Medical and Dental staff in England 1991-2001.
(a) 2001 figure.

### Table 5.3.27
### Clinical oncologists: consultant and non-career grades:
### UK establishment (posts) 2002

| Country | Grade | Substantive | Vacant | Grand total |
|---|---|---|---|---|
| England | Associate Specialist | 12 | | 12 |
| | Clinical Assistant | 7 | | 7 |
| | Consultant | 336 | 19 | 362 |
| | Consultant (+ Prof) | 4 | | 4 |
| | Consultant (+snr lecturer) | 8 | 1 | 9 |
| | Staff Grade | 20 | 2 | 23 |
| | Total | 387 | 22 | 417 |
| Scotland | Consultant | 41 | 1 | 42 |
| | Consultant (+ Prof) | 3 | | 3 |
| | Consultant (+snr lecturer) | 1 | | 1 |
| | Staff Grade | | 1 | 1 |
| | Total | 45 | 2 | 47 |
| UK Total | | 477 | 24 | 510 |

Source: UK RT Survey 2002, A multidisciplinary survey of radiotherapy services in the UK at 4 June 2002.

In Scotland, *Action for Change* recognised the need for and promised more key staff in order to minimise delays in investigation, diagnosis and treatment of cancer. November 2001 saw the announcement of £10 million extra resources for NHS recruitment that were to result in 28 more cancer specialists as well as extra nurses and radiographers being employed in Scotland.[208] The National Implementation investment plans detail £2.3 million (2001-2002-2003) for additional investigation and diagnostic staff 'including at least 13 consultants, 3 clinical nurse specialists, 9 nurses, 17 radiographers, 5 endoscopists and 18 other support staff.[209] Over the same period, a further £3.5 million has been invested in improving cancer treatment and care; this amount represents 'at least 21 consultants, 34 clinical nurse specialists, 17 nurses, 5 radiographers, 4 pharmacists and 25 other support staff.[210] A further allocation of £0.9 million has been made for extra staff and technology including 4 consultants and 4 radiographers.

The announcement of these extra funds to treat cancer was overshadowed by a *BMJ* report which highlighted

problems at Scotland's biggest cancer treatment centre—
('The Beatson'), after the resignation of four consultants
between November 2001 and February 2002 and 'claims
that the service is at breaking point' (these problems were
already well-known in Scotland).[211] The Beatson Oncology
Centre in Glasgow treats 60 per cent of all Scottish cancer
cases, but staff have been concerned that resources have not
kept pace with extra workload; in a 1998 report 'the Royal
College of Radiologists recommended that consultant
oncologists should only see 315 new patients a year [but],
some of the oncologists at the Beatson are seeing twice that
number ... The centre should have 11 linear accelerators
(see below) to treat the population it services, but it only
has six.'[212] Accordingly, waiting times are longer than is
recommended and doctors warn that those delays lead to
poorer outcomes for some patients.[213] Following that report,
in February 2002 an extra £10 million (on top of the £40
million previously promised) was committed for the implementation of *Action for Change*. The Beatson Oncology
Centre was to receive £2 million of this additional investment.[214] The annual report 2002 of *Action for Change* tells
us that more than 50 additional staff are now employed at
the Beatson.

### Sub-specialisation

Sub-specialisation has become more prevalent amid
evidence that it leads to improved patient outcomes.
Evidence in England shows some variation between trusts.
Table 5.3.28 shows the number of surgeons and physicians
on agreed sub-specialisation lists. We have not found
similar data for Scotland.

## Table 5.3.28
### The number of surgeons and physicians on agreed sub-specialisation lists

| Type of cancer | Where there are agreed lists of sub-specialists, how many doctors are on each list? | | | | |
|---|---|---|---|---|---|
| | Number of trusts/ hospitals with each number: | | | | |
| | 1 doctor | 2 | 3 | 4 | 5 or more |
| Breast | 4 | 7 | 7 | 1 | 0 |
| Colon | 3 | 6 | 2 | 0 | 2 |
| Ovary | 4 | 7 | 0 | 0 | 0 |
| Leukaemia | 2 | 6 | 2 | 0 | 0 |
| Lung | 3 | 4 | 2 | 1 | 1 |
| Malignant melanoma | 1 | 5 | 1 | 0 | 1 |
| Pancreas | 3 | 3 | 1 | 1 | 1 |
| Prostate | 3 | 6 | 3 | 0 | 0 |

Source: CHI/AC report of site visits: 16 hospitals/trusts within nine networks.
CHI/Audit Commission, 2001, Supporting Data 6, Sub Specialisation, Table 6

## Diagnostic and Treatment Equipment

Following diagnosis, curative cancer treatment may involve surgery, radiotherapy, chemotherapy, or a combination of the three. Precise information on cancer location and size is usually obtained by CT and MRI scanning. To avoid delays in the commencement of treatment there must be an adequate number of available scanners. Treatment with radiotherapy is 'an extremely important modality in the management of cancer'.[215] It is used to kill tumour cells and may be part of curative treatment or may be used to reduce symptoms from advanced disease (palliative radiotherapy).[216] In either case, in order to provide timely treatment there must be a sufficient number of machines.[217] Hughes and the ARD Team at the OECD link the UK's poor cancer performance to rationing—or what it politely calls 'supply-side constraints'.[218] For example, one of their charts correlates the five-year survival rate with the availability of the mammography machines used for breast-cancer screening. There are few machines in the UK compared with other OECD countries and outcomes are poor. In relation to breast cancer, Hughes highlights the fact that: 'assessing performance is a complex task, which would involve multivariate analysis of variations in survival; however, the data available to us for international comparison is very limited.' Nevertheless, their team attempted to examine the impact of technological inputs on various outcomes, including recommended treatment rates, screening rates and survival rates.[219] Hughes states that 'no conclusions can be drawn' from their study, and that 'survival rates do not seem to depend on the availability of state-of-the-art technology',[220] but posited that it was likely that countries with a higher proportion of cancers at an advanced stage might be 'experiencing lack of access to mammography screening and other diagnostic services—whether it is the supply of machines or human resources that cause delays in diagnosis' (see Table 5.3.29 for availability of such equipment).[221] Although these findings should not be accepted uncritically, it is likely that they apply to both Scotland and England.

Similarly, the OECD has compared five-year survival with the availability of radiotherapy machines (generally LinAc machines [external beam machines]) used to treat cancer. The UK has fewer machines than other countries and a worse survival rate. As the report says, the UK 'clearly stands out', a conclusion suggesting that inadequate staff and facilities have caused the poor survival rate.[222] The OECD also compares death rates within six months of diagnosis. Again the UK has a higher rate of death within six months, suggesting that cancers are more advanced when detected. This is likely to be because of the inadequate number of staff and the shortage of equipment for early detection. This means that the NHS in both England and Scotland has been failing to do one of the most important things a highly centralised system ought to be capable of: organising a system of universal screening to ensure early detection.

England and Scotland are well below average in the supply of radiation facilities (see Tables 5.3.29 - 5.3.31 for UK and international comparisons of the availability of such equipment).[223] But things have changed since Calman-Hine; acknowledging England's poor international standing, the *NHS Plan Implementation Programme* pledged that the

English regions must make progress to the *NHS Plan* targets that by 2004 there will be 50 new MRI scanners, 200 new CT scanners, 80 new liquid cytology units and 45 new linear accelerators.[224] The NHS has invested in some new equipment. Since April 2000, '39 new MRI scanners, 55 linear accelerators, 119 CT scanners and over 450 items of breast screening equipment' have been delivered.[225]

There are 20 linear accelerators in Scotland's five cancer centres.[226] *Cancer Scenarios* called for an increase in this number to 31 by 2010—based on the assumption there should be five LinAcs per million population. *Cancer Scenarios* also called for more CT and MRI scanners; between 2001 and 2003, £3.9 million was to be spent on vital machinery such as MRI, CT scanners, endoscopy, ultrasound, mammography, and pathology equipment.

In 2001, CHI and the Audit Commission reported inequity in the distribution of LinAc machines in England and of their use—which affects both costs and waiting times.[227] There is also a variation in the working hours of such machines; 'for instance, over two-thirds of all machines are used only between 9 a.m. and 5 p.m. on weekdays'.[228] The same uneven patterns of distribution and of use are seen in Scotland.[229]

Of course, the diagnostic and therapeutic machinery discussed above must be operated by well-qualified staff (see Tables 5.3.32 and 5.3.33). There are serious shortages of radiographers and radiotherapy physicists (who operate LinAcs) in both England and Scotland. Between 1992 and 1997 the number of radiographers in Scotland decreased by 3.9 per cent overall, despite an increase in use of LinAcs by 4.6 per cent.[230] This compares less favourably with the UK overall, which showed a 17 per cent increase, in line with the increase in workload.[231] However, between 1997 and 2001 there has been a steady increase in radiographers in Scotland and England, with no significant difference in the rate of increase between the two countries. The change in staffing levels in Scotland and England between 1997 and 2001 is given below.

## Table 5.3.29

### Radiation treatment equipment per million population (pmp)

| Country | Radiation Treatment Equipment (LAF) pmp | Number of LinAcs (LAF) | MRI Scanners Rate (LAF) pmp | CT Scanners Rate (LAF) pmp |
|---|---|---|---|---|
| England | 3.8 | 189 (a) | 3.46 (171) | 5.66 (280) |
| Scotland | 3.0 | 20 (b) | 3.13 (16) | 5.6 (c) |
| OECD Average | 6.6 | N/A | 6.4 | 16.8 |

*Source*: NHSScotland, *Cancer Scenarios*. OECD *Health Data 2002*. National Cancer Services Analysis Team, NHS Executive (North West) website (www.cancernw.org.uk/ accessed 18 March 2003. And Royal College of Radiologists *et al*., UK RT Survey 2002, A multidisciplinary survey of radiotherapy services in the UK at 4 June 2002.

*Note*: England figures for 2000; Scotland for 2000; OECD for 1999.
(a) 182 of these 189 were working in June 2002.
(b) We are told by the Scottish Executive that this figure is due to rise to 24 within the next year or two (personal comments from the ISD).
(c) Figure for 2002, estimated from Scottish Executive, *Coronary Heart Disease and Stroke: Strategy for Scotland*, 2002 (Appendix 4).

## Table 5.3.30

### Megavoltage radiation treatment equipment in clinical use at 04.06.2002, per million population (pmp)

| Country | Catchment Populations | Machines | | | Machines per million | | |
|---|---|---|---|---|---|---|---|
| | | Linacs | Cobalts | Megavoltage | Linacs | Cobalts | Megavoltage |
| England | 47,321,918 | 168 | 7 | 171.5 | 3.55 | 0.15 | 3.62 |
| Scotland | 4,998,256 | 17 | 0 | 17.0 | 3.40 | 0.00 | 3.40 |
| UK | 56,830,155 | 199 | 8 | 203.0 | 3.50 | 0.14 | 3.57 |

*Source*: UK RT Survey 2002, A multidisciplinary survey of radiotherapy services in the UK at 4 June 2002.
*Notes*: number of megavoltage machines = number of Linacs + 0.5 (number of cobalt machines).
Populations calculated from 1991 Census Population Data.

### Table 5.3.31
### Healthcare technology resources

| Country Characteristic | Denmark | England | France | Germany | Netherlands | Switzerland | Scotland | UK | USA |
|---|---|---|---|---|---|---|---|---|---|
| CT scanners per million | 10.9 | 5.66 | 9.6 | 17.1 | 7.2 (92) | 18.5 | 5.6 | 3.6 | 13.6 |
| MRIs per million | 6.6 (00) | 3.49 | 2.5 (97) | 6.2 (97) | 3.9 | 13.0 | 3.13 | 3.9 (99) | 8.1 |
| Radiation treatment Equipment per million | N/A | 3.8 | 7.6 (97) | 4.7 (96) | N/A | 5.0 (98) | 3.0 | 3.5 (98) | 3.8 (92) |
| Public investment in med facilities as % TEH | 2.8 | N/A | 2.4 | 2.6 | N/A | 2.7 | N/A | 2.5 | 0.4 |
| + per capita PPPs | 68 | N/A | 50 | 63 | N/A | 76 | N/A | 39 | 15 |

Source: Civitas commissioned research. NHSScotland, Cancer Scenarios, p. 307; OECD, Health Data 2002.
National Cancer Services Analysis Team, NHS Executive (North West) website (www.cancernw.org.uk/ accessed 18 March 2003.

## Table 5.3.32
## Number of radiographers

| Country | 1997 | 1998 | 1999 | 2000 | 2001 | % change |
|---------|------|------|------|------|------|----------|
| England | 9,910 | 10,190 | 10,370 | 10,480 | 10,650 | +7.5 |
| Scotland | 1,360 | 1,368 | 1,419 | 1,408 | 1,466 | +7.8 |

*Source:* England: NHS HCHS non-medical staff; Scotland: ISD

## Table 5.3.33
## Therapy radiographers:
## UK establishment and occupancy (WTE), 2002

| Country | Substantive | Grand total | % vacant |
|---------|-------------|-------------|----------|
| England | 737.81 | 796.61 | 6.3 |
| Scotland | 83.7 | 64.2 | 10.1 |
| UK | 882.85 | 958.15 | 6.3 |

*Source:* UK RT Survey 2002, A multidisciplinary survey of radiotherapy services in the UK at 4 June 2002

## Table 5.3.34
## Number of consultant radiologists

| Country | 1997 | 1998 | 1999 | 2000 | 2001 | % change |
|---------|------|------|------|------|------|----------|
| England | 1,470 | 1,510 | 1,540 | 1,620 | 1,680 | +14.3 |
| Scotland | 192 | 192 | 199 | 205 | 203 | +5.7 |

*Source:* NHS Statistical Bulletin 2002/4

Shortages in the number of radiographers, while a major factor in the low rates of treatment, are quicker to remedy than shortages in trained radiologists, who require considerably more time and investment to train. Improvements in technology and changes in treatment have meant that the role of radiologists has changed dramatically in the past 25 years. In addition to radiography and complex imaging procedures, radiologists now contribute to patient management and therapeutic procedures. Here too there is a dearth of qualified consultants, who have traditionally delivered clinical radiology in the UK. In Scotland in 2001, 11.5 per cent of consultant radiologist posts were unfilled, and in England in March 2002 eight per cent of posts were unfilled.[232] The Royal College of Radiologists has suggested that there needs to be an increase in the number of consultants from the current level of 1,940 to 3,300 to meet existing workload requirements.[233]

## Cancer Screening in England and Scotland

### Breast cancer screening

Screening has a direct effect on early detection and the number of diagnosed cases and affects survival.[234] The progression of the disease at diagnosis determines the type of treatment that can be offered, the response to treatment, and survival chances.[235] It is apparent that countries such as the USA with high breast cancer incidence also tend to have higher survival rates; it is likely that screening reveals minor cancers, many of which are unlikely to result in death, boosting both incidence and survival rates. In 2001 a Swedish study reported on in the *BMJ* found that screening with mammography reduces deaths from breast cancer by nearly two thirds.[236] A number of studies have contradicted findings on the efficacy of mammography, however, and the International Agency for Research on Cancer (IARC) of the World Health Organisation has concluded that mammography of women aged 50-69 years old reduces breast cancer mortality by 35 per cent.[237] Accordingly, by 2004, all women in England aged 50-70 are to be invited for breast screening.[238]

Table 5.3.35 shows breast screening data from Scotland and England. In England since 1995, the number of women screened per year has risen by c. 15 per cent, and the number of those with cancer detected following screening has risen by c. 45 per cent.[239] At 69.8 per cent, screening coverage in England had been rising for six years from 63.9 per cent in 1994-95 towards the Government's target of 70 per cent, but represents a fall from the 2001/02 figures (70.2 per cent), while at 75.6 per cent, uptake during 2001-02 was slightly lower than it has been since 1994-95 (77.4 per cent).[240] Coverage of the standard target age-group varied significantly between NHS England regional office areas; from 57.9 per cent in London to over 74 per cent in Trent.[241]

## Table 5.3.35
## Breast screening in Scotland and England

| | Scotland 98/99-00/01 | England 2001-02 |
|---|---|---|
| Coverage: % women aged 50-64 screened in previous three years *(i.e less than three years since last test)* | 73.2% | 69.8% |
| % of women aged 53-64 screened in previous three years *(i.e. less than three years since last test)* | 74.3% | 75.9% |
| Uptake: % of women aged 50-64 invited for screening who were scanned | 73.6%* | 75.6% |
| Number of women (all ages) scanned | 133,302 | c. 1.3 million |
| Cancer detection rate per 1,000 screened women aged 50-64 | | |
|     Prevalent | 5.9 | 4.5 West Midlands<br>4.7 London<br>6.1 Trent |
|     Incident | 5.1 | 4.3 West Midlands<br>4.5 London<br>4.3 Trent |
| Standardised detection ratio | | |
|     Prevalent | 1.47 | 1.35 West Midlands<br>1.25 London<br>1.67 Trent |
|     Incident | 1.27 | 1.08 West Midlands<br>1.12 London<br>1.06 Trent |
| Subsequent diagnoses of cancer | | |
| Ages 45+ | 965 (all ages) | 8,545 (all ages) |
| Ages 50-64 | | 7,009 (2000-01) |

* refers to data for 1999/2000

*Sources*: Scotland – Scottish Breast Screening Programme; DoH, *Building on Experience, Breast Screening Programme Annual Review 2002*, NHS, 2002.
England – 'Return KC62 (from the 84 screening units)' and 'Return KC63 (from Health Authorities)' Department of Health, *Breast Screening Programme England: Bulletin 2001-02 February 2003*; Department of Health, *Breast Screening Programme England: Bulletin 2000-01*, 2002, pp. 1-5.

*Notes*: The coverage of the SP is the proportion of women resident who have had a test with a recorded result at least once in the previous three years. The uptake of the SP is the proportion of women invited for screening for whom a screening test result is recorded. Prevalent screening is that of women being screened for the first time within the breast screening programme. Incident screening is that of women previously screened within the breast screening programme.

Of the slightly under 1.5 million 50-64 year-olds invited to screening, 1.3 million (75.3 per cent) were screened at one of the 84 screening units in England. When analysed by screening unit, uptake rates vary by region, with seven of the eight lowest (below 70 per cent) being found in London.[242] Roughly four per cent of those screened were aged between 45 and 49, while eight per cent were 65 or over.[243]

The cancer detection rate in England in 2001-02 was 6.7 per 1,000 women screened. The incident round rate rose from 5.5 to 5.9 cases per 1,000 screened (2001-02). Meanwhile, the prevalent round detection rate rose from 6.1 (in 1999-00), to 6.6 per cent (in 2001-02). The statistics show that the detection rate varies significantly with age: at ages 45-49 (5.1 per 1,000), ages 50-59 (5.9 per 1,000), ages 60-64 (7.4 per cent per 1,000), and age 65 or over (11.2 per 1,000); emphasising how important it is that screening be readily available to older age-groups.[244]

*Table 5.3.36*
*Breast screening programme: test status and coverage*
*by age, 31 March 2002, England*

| Age at test | Number of women resident | Coverage (less than three years since last test) % |
|---|---|---|
| 60-64 | 1,228.6 | 75.2 |
| 65-69 | 1,134.5 | 35.1 |
| 70 | 219.8 | 14.1 |
| 71-74 | 852.5 | 7.3 |
| 75 and over | 2,408.3 | 1.1 |

*Source*: Department of Health, *Breast Screening Programme England: Bulletin 2001-02*, February 2003, Form KC63

It is not surprising that the OECD ARD Team found some evidence that older women (70+) may not be receiving a regular mammogram. In Canada 65-70 per cent of women aged 50-60 report receiving a mammogram in the preceding two years. This percentage falls to 44-49 for those 70 and over. Only 3.2 per cent of those 70+ in the UK are screened.[245] See Tables 5.3.36 and 5.3.37 for recent evidence.

## Table 5.3.37

### Breast screening programme: women screened by age and outcome 2001-02

| Age | Number of women screened | | Referred for assessment (%) | | Cancer detected total rate per 1,000 screened | |
|---|---|---|---|---|---|---|
| | Scotland | England | Scotland | England | Scotland | England |
| 50-54 | 46,195 | 441,186 | 11.0/4.9 | 6.8 | 5.9/3.1 | 5.7 |
| 55-59 | 38,421 | 380,718 | 10.0/4.9 | 4.5 | 6.3/5.3 | 6.2 |
| 60-64 | 34,977 | 300,440 | 8.4/6.2 | 4.2 | 9.5/6.2 | 7.4 |
| 65-69 | 823 | 78,910 | 3.7/6.3 | 4.6 | 0.0/0.0 | 9.9 |
| 70 & over | 9 | 32,064 | 0.0/0.0 | 5.8 | 0.0/0.0 | 14.5 |

*Sources*: Department of Health, *Breast Screening Programme England: Bulletin 2001-02*, February 2003 Form KC62, Tables 7a and 9a. Scottish figures for referral for assessment: first number refers to those attending screening for the first time, while the second is for those attending a routine subsequent screen. Similarly the figures for cancers detected are divided for Scotland between first and subsequent screens. Scottish figures are for invasive cancers, while English figures also include non-invasive cancers.

Screening coverage in Scotland is slightly lower than that in England. The percentage of all those invited to screening who attend in Scotland has increased a little from around 71 per cent to 73 per cent (1990-2001)—though these figures hide significant variation between those at different points of Carstairs' Deprivation Category: those on the lowest point of the scale had a take-up of c. 51 per cent while 78 per cent (1996/7 figures) of those on the top of the scale attended.[246] Similar deprivation data were not available for England. As in England, there are also significant geographical variations in screening take-up (high rates are seen in Grampian (83 per cent), Shetland (86.9 per cent) and Orkney (88.5 per cent). Low rates are seen in the industrial central belt (Glasgow 66.2 per cent, Lanarkshire 69.3 per cent, Lothian 69.7 per cent). In the year ending March 2001, 5.7 invasive cancers were detected per 1,000 women screened. In 2000/2001 85.5 per cent of breast cancers were diagnosed pre-operatively—up from 67.7 per cent in 1996/97.

Comparing Scotland and England, certain patterns of screening can be observed: Scotland always has the highest recall rate for the first screening round.[247]

OECD Health has highlighted the UK's poor record in breast cancer screening, and drawn the rather cautious conclusion that 'given the restrictions in terms of the availability of qualified medical staff, screening and radiation treatment equipment, financial constraints in terms of treatment may have had an impact on outcomes'.[248]

*Cervical cancer screening*

As the *NHS Cancer Plan* for England states: 'Cervical screening identifies abnormalities which, if left untreated *may* [original emphasis] develop into cancer.'[249] Smears are taken by GPs, practice nurses, or at a community clinic. A referral to colposcopy may follow. English policy is that eligible women (the target is those aged 20-64) should be screened every three to five years.[250] Similarly, cervical screening in Scotland is well established and available to women aged 20-60 once every three years.[251] Those over 60

can be screened on request and those with previous abnormalities continue to be invited. Scottish Health Statistics
for 1999 showed that cervical screening prevents up to 250
cases of cervical cancer each year.[252] *Action for Change*
announced that a new IT system was due to be developed by
late spring 2003, to improve the first invitation and recall
procedures for cervical screening in Scotland.[253]

### *Table 5.3.38*
### *Cervical cancer screening by country,*
### *latest available year*

| Indicator | Scotland | England |
|---|---|---|
| Coverage* (target range)† | 86.5% | 81.6% (a) |
| Number of women invited 2000-01 (T3,4,5,6) | | |
|     All age-groups | N/A | 4,095,057 |
|     (ages 20-64) | N/A | 3,971,300 |
| Number of women screened 2000-01 (T7+T8) | | |
|     All age-groups | N/A | 3,633,479 |
|     Target range | 331,218‡ | 3,522,403 |
| Result of test negative 2000-01 (T7+T8) | | |
|     Target range | 92.0% | 92.1 % |

Sources: Department of Health, *England: Cervical Screening Programme England:
Bulletin 2002/21*, October 2002.
Scotland: Cancer Research UK: Cervical Screening – UK, from Cervical Screening
Programme[254]

Notes:
* England: less than five years since last adequate test. Scotland: less than five and a
half years since last adequate test.
† For Scotland this is 20-60, for England 20-64
‡ Excludes Lothian. Data unavailable.
(a) Although target range is 20-64, English coverage figures are for women aged 25-64.

As with breast screening, screening coverage rates vary
geographically; in England, at 75.9 per cent, those in
London are lowest and those in Trent (84.2) highest,[255]
while in Scotland, although the mean rate is higher, the
range of variation is similar (Greater Glasgow has the
lowest rate at 82.3 per cent, Orkney has the highest rate at
93 per cent). Again, perhaps unsurprisingly, the number of
positive tests falls up to the ages-group 60-64, at which
point it rises again, to 91.9 for those aged 75 and over.[256]

*Breast cancer treatment and radiation therapy in England and Scotland*

According to Johnston and McDermott, it has been shown that there are variations in treatment geographically in the UK, in breast cancer, with respect to patients who obtain breast conservation, those patients who are offered breast reconstruction, and those patients who are given post operative chemotherapy and radiotherapy.[257] Unfortunately, we have not found sufficient comparable evidence on breast cancer treatment and radiation therapy in England and Scotland. However, recent international studies allow comparison of the UK, with its poor survival rates, with other developed countries. Some of this evidence is presented here.

There are three established breast cancer treatments: mastectomy; breast-conserving surgery (BCS); and breast-conserving surgery with post-operative radiation therapy (known as RT after BCS).[258] Since 1985 it has been accepted that RT after BCS has produced a similar survival rate to mastectomy for women diagnosed with early-stage breast cancer, whilst avoiding the disfiguring effect of whole breast removal. Nevertheless, rates of BCS as opposed to mastectomy in those aged over 40 vary considerably across countries.[259] In all countries examined by the OECD's ARD team, treatments varied with increasing age—fewer women 70 years and over received BCS. But the degree of variation in treatments also differs sharply. Patients in Belgium, Canada, France, Italy, Norway and the US received lower levels of BCS in older age-groups. In (tax-financed) Sweden and the UK the difference was more stark. Those aged 80+ in Sweden and the UK were half as likely as those aged 70-79, to receive BCS in 1994-5 (see Table 5.3.39).[260]

Treatment patterns in the UK are singled out for comment by the OECD; both mastectomy and BCS rates for older women are very low compared to other countries. Hughes shows that mastectomy rates tend to rise with age (at least to age 79). However, the UK shows a rate of 11 per cent of those 80+ receiving mastectomy, with the average for the eight countries studied being nearly 49 per cent. The

UK also has a very low BCS rate for those aged 80+ of only 14 per cent, compared to the average of 28 per cent (see Table 5.3.39).[261]

*Table 5.3.39*
**Women receiving breast conserving surgery as a**
**percentage of women diagnosed with breast cancer**

| Country/Year | Age | | | | | |
|---|---|---|---|---|---|---|
| | 40-49 | 50-59 | 60-64 | 65-69 | 70-79 | 80+ |
| Belgium (1997) | 67 | 69 | 64 | 59 | 51 | 44 |
| Canada (1995) | 45 | 45 | 42 | 42 | 38 | 29 |
| Canada (Manitoba (1995-98) | 71 | 75 | 67 | 71 | 62 | 54 |
| Canada (Ontario) (1995) | 53 | 56 | 56 | 53 | 51 | 44 |
| France (1997) | 66 | 71 | 65 | 65 | 53 | 39 |
| Italy (1990-91) | 38 | 26 | 31 | 26 | 21 | 21 |
| Norway (1995) | 26 | 30 | 19 | 17 | 13 | 23 |
| Sweden (1994) (a) | 49 | 51 | 43 | Na | 32 | 13 |
| UK – England (1995) | 56 | 56 | 55 | 45 | 34 | 14 |
| USA (1995-97) (b) | N/A | 54 | 52 | 50 | 48 | 43 |

*Source*: OECD, ARD Team, Breast Cancer Disease Report, 2002 (Table 2, p. 18).
(a) Swedish estimates for 60-64 years reflect 60-69 years.
(b) US estimates are not available for 40-49 years.

The use of RT after BCS varies widely from 57 per cent of those receiving BCS in Italy, to 90 per cent and 93 per cent in Belgium and France respectively. Variation in RT by age is notable in all countries; there is a sharp decline for those over 70. A drop at ages 70-79 occurs in Canada, Italy, Sweden and the UK. However, in Belgium, France and the US patients in that group receive similar treatment to those in younger groups.[262]

As part of the ARD study, the OECD team also examined the effect regulatory and economic incentives may have on the treatment of breast cancer care and survival across 13 OECD countries.[263] Specifically, they explored the relationship between prevalence of BCS, RT after BCS, and mastectomy for breast cancer and variations in economic and regulatory factors in the healthcare delivery and financing systems. Delays in radiation therapy that could be linked to resource availability and productive efficiency have been highlighted in Canada, Norway, Sweden and the UK—all tax-funded systems.[264] While Hughes did not directly ask the question, it is reasonable to draw attention to the fact that certain system features are more associated with social insurance schemes, while others are found commonly in tax-based systems; i.e. Scotland and England.

Again, the payment mechanism also may have had an impact on medical outcomes. The ARD team also note that those countries using global budgets (Norway, Sweden, Canada and the UK [England and Scotland]) generally have BCS rates lower than 50 per cent. Countries with DRG or fee-for-service payment systems had higher rates.[265] Flexible payment mechanisms as seen in France, Belgium and the US allow each patient to be seen as a source of income, giving more incentive to refer.[266] Other studies have also found that reimbursement practices themselves affect treatments provided. In the US it has been found that higher reimbursement levels for BCS lead to greater BCS use.[267]

Hughes and the ARD team conclude that better cancer care performance is achieved through a mix of population-based breast cancer screening programmes, combined with treatment protocols that follow the most recent clinical guidelines, without being unnecessarily limited by economic constraints.[268]

### Lung cancer treatment

Surgical resection offers the best chance of cure and is the recognised ideal treatment for stage I or II non-small-cell lung cancer sufferers. In Scotland surgical resection rates are similar to those in England: they lie at about ten per cent.[269] These rates are low compared to other developed countries. For example, resection rates of 24 per cent and 25 per cent have been reported in Dutch and American patients.[270] According to Janssen-Heijnen *et al.* of the EUROCARE II working group the proportion of patients receiving surgery was relatively high in Switzerland, France and the Netherlands, and low in the UK.[271]

Patients who could potentially be saved by resection are not being offered the treatment. The lack of appropriate treatment has been blamed quite simply on a shortage of specialist thoracic surgeons; there are 31 purely thoracic surgeons in the England and Wales. Professor Tom Treasure, one of the authors of a 2001 report, said that the problem may stem from the fact that lung cancer has not been given the same emphasis as other cancers as it is perceived as a self-inflicted disease.[272]

Janssen-Heijnen et al. suggest that the lower survival rates for patients with lung cancer in Scotland and England may be partly explained by poor access to specialised care. The number of consultants is lower than in most other European countries, the percentage of histological verification was considerably lower,[273] (it was 61 per cent in Scotland and 58 per cent in England compared to 91 per cent in Finland, 82 per cent in Germany, 99 per cent in Switzerland and 95 per cent in France) and the proportion of patients receiving 'curative' treatment was also much lower.[274] Studies suggest this proportion is slightly lower in England compared to Scotland (between 47 per cent and 48 per cent received no active treatment in England, compared to 42 per cent receiving no treatment in Scotland).[275]

Janssen-Heijnen et al. found that the proportion of patients with small-cell lung cancer receiving chemotherapy was highest in France, the Netherlands and Switzerland, and lowest in the UK.[276] Some variation has been noted between studies carried out in England and Scotland. The percentage of patients receiving any chemotherapy in Scotland in the Gregor et al 1995 study was 62.7 per cent. In the Melling et al. Yorkshire study it was 55.1 per cent.[277]

### Summary

Our findings on health outcomes and standard treatments can be summarised as follows:

*Health outcomes*

- Life expectancy is lower for Scottish men and women than for the English
- Infant mortality is almost identical in England and Scotland

- Incidence of major cancers is (tends to be) higher in Scotland
- Prevalence of CHD is slightly higher in Scotland
- Incidence of stroke is higher in Scotland
- Mortality from major cancers is higher in Scotland
- Mortality from CHD is higher in Scotland
- Mortality from stroke is higher in Scotland
- One- and five-year survival from all cancers is slightly better in England. However, Scotland appears to perform fractionally better than England for some cancers (most notably for prostate cancer) and fractionally worse for others (including cervical cancer). Overall, English men seem to fare slightly less well than Scots for the main cancers we explored, while English women appear to have very slightly better survival than the Scots
- There is significant geographical variation in cancer incidence, mortality and survival in both countries.

*Standard treatments*

- Standard treatment rates we have explored tend to be higher in Scotland
- Rates of CABG are higher in Scotland
- PTCA rates have been higher in Scotland for some years but are now roughly the same as those in England
- Treatment in specialist stroke units is more common in Scotland (65 per cent of patients as opposed to 49 per cent)
- Breast and cervical screening programmes cover more people in Scotland.
- The percentage of histological verification for lung cancer patients is slightly higher in Scotland, as the percentage of those receiving curative treatments
- Expenditure on statin prescriptions per capita is higher in Scotland.

# 6

# Discussion

# Benedict Irvine

In a report for the Social Exclusion Unit in 2000, Dr
Jennifer Dixon noted that there is little consensus about
what constitutes a 'quality' indicator in health care. A
variety of information can be used: structures or inputs (e.g.
measuring numbers of staff, funding), processes (e.g. GP
consultation rates, hospital admission rates) and outcomes
(e.g. survival rates, death rates).[1] In the course of this study
we have collected data on inputs, with details of processes
and outcomes where they were available. Our findings can
be summarised as follows:

## On Funding

- Scotland spends significantly more than England on
  healthcare
- Funding is predominantly public in both countries, but
  private expenditure is significantly higher in England
- Taxation is the major source of healthcare funds in both
  countries
- Expenditure per capita on family medical services is
  slightly higher in Scotland
- Hospital care expenditure per capita and per household
  is higher in Scotland.

## On Resources

- Healthcare resources are predominantly publicly owned
  and managed in both countries
- There is more private provision in England

- The NHS is the largest employer in both England and Scotland
- There are fewer doctors, dentists, nurses, and midwives per capita in England than Scotland
- There are more GPs per capita in Scotland (lists sizes are smaller in Scotland)
- The number of elderly (those over 65 and those over 75) on GP lists is lower on average in Scotland
- There are more consultant cardiologists per head in Scotland
- There are slightly more specialist and medical oncologists per head in Scotland
- There are fewer acute beds per capita in England than Scotland
- There are fewer available beds per medical, dental, and nursing staff in England
- There are fewer radiotherapy/diagnostic (MRI/CT/ LinAc) machines per capita in Scotland
- The number of specialist stroke units per million is significantly higher in Scotland
- There is significant geographical variation in resource provision in both countries.

### *On Activity*

- There are more finished consultant episodes (FCEs)per medical and dental staff in England
- FCEs/discharges and deaths per bed are significantly higher in England
- Bed occupancy rates are similar, though higher in England
- Average length of stay is longer in Scotland
- Total attendances (per 1,000) at hospital outpatient clinics are higher in Scotland.

### *On Population and Environmental Inputs*

- Alcohol consumption is higher in Scotland than in England
- Tobacco consumption is higher in Scotland
- Diet (measured by fruit, vegetable and fat consumption) in Scotland is poorer than that in England
- There is little difference in overweight or obesity between England and Scotland. The only group in which any significant difference was revealed was Scottish women aged 16-24, who showed greater prevalence of overweight and obesity
- Rates of exercise in Scotland are often lower than those in England (age-group dependent)
- Blood cholesterol levels are higher in England
- Hypertension is more prevalent in England
- Systolic and diastolic blood pressure is lower in Scotland over all ages and both sexes
- Income inequality is less pronounced in Scotland
- But there is greater income-related health inequality in Scotland
- There is significant geographical variation in services provided in both countries
- Screening programmes cover more in Scotland.

### *On Health Outcomes*

- Life expectancy is lower for Scottish men and women than for the English
- Infant mortality is almost identical in England and Scotland
- Incidence of major cancers tends to be higher in Scotland
- Prevalence of CHD is slightly higher in Scotland
- Incidence of stroke is higher in Scotland
- Alcohol related mortality is higher in Scotland

- Mortality from major cancers is higher in Scotland
- Mortality from CHD is higher in Scotland
- Mortality from stroke is higher in Scotland
- Mortality for Scottish women of working age is a particular concern
- One- and five- year survival from all cancers is slightly better in England. However, Scotland appears to perform fractionally better than England for some cancers (most notably for prostate cancer) and fractionally worse for others (including cervical cancer). Overall, English men seem to fare slightly less well than Scots for the main cancers we explored, while English women appear to have very slightly better survival than the Scots
- There is significant geographical variation in incidence, mortality and survival in both countries. (For the years 1995-97, Glasgow City had the lowest life expectancy at birth of any local authority in the UK.)
- Comparing Scotland and England risks masking the poor position of the UK in an international context.

### On Standard Treatments

- Rates of activity we have explored tend to be higher in Scotland
- Rates of CABG are higher in Scotland
- PTCA rates have been higher in Scotland for some years but are now roughly the same as those in England
- Breast and Cervical screening programmes cover more people in Scotland
- The percentage of histological verification for lung cancer patients is slightly higher in Scotland, as is the percentage of those receiving curative treatments
- Treatment in specialist stroke units is more common in Scotland (65 per cent of patients as opposed to 49 per cent)
- Expenditure on statin prescriptions per capita is higher in Scotland.

As for most comparative research, these simplified findings are subject to numerous caveats regarding the quality and comparability of data, differences between sexes and regions, and the fact that, though both predominantly public in nature, there are differing provider structures in England and Scotland. Nevertheless, some trends are clear. The objective of this report was to make an assessment of the funding, quality and performance of NHS health services in England and Scotland. Unfortunately, the scope of our research does not permit in-depth analysis of the causal relationship between resources, funding and outcomes. Instead we observe trends and pose some questions.

### On Funding

We know health funding has been higher in Scotland for many years and that Scotland spends tax revenue at a level to which England aspires. It is implicit in our hypothesis that the desired increase in funds, in England, will, in coming years, be from taxation—at least while Gordon Brown is in charge at the Treasury.

While scholars struggle to make a connection between spending and outcomes, OECD researchers and Dominghetti and Quaglia have found that increased expenditure leads to improved health outcomes.[2] Total expenditure on healthcare per capita is correlated with health status.[3] Plural funding systems spend more on healthcare. A cluster of consistently higher indicators is found among those countries spending $1,700 PPP per capita, or more.[4] Beyond that threshold, one does not find a clear positive correlation between performance and increased expenditure.[5] From what we have found, Scotland seems to be an exception—a country that spends more but perhaps does not benefit from improved outcomes. Bearing in mind that public expenditure as a percentage of total expenditure on health is higher in Scotland and England, we can pose the question: 'if the extra per capita spending in Scotland had been from another funding source, would outcomes have improved?' The received wisdom in Scotland, and for many English observers, is that social deprivation is the explanation (see below); in part it is, but the methods by which resources are raised and subsequently distributed may also be important factors.

## On Resources

Despite the current policy, which is increasing health spending very rapidly in England, health systems subject to central political management tend to limit the availability of resources, especially the number of doctors, in the belief that medical demand is 'supplier induced' and has little bearing on medical outcomes. However, more recent research shows that there is an optimal spending level that varies over time, typically increasing with per capita income. The availability of medical resources has a beneficial impact on medical outcomes.[6] Consequently, a well-organised healthcare system will allow the availability of resources to vary over time to meet both professionally-defined medical needs as well as consumer-defined medical demands.

The supply of advanced diagnostic and treatment technology such as MRI and CT scanners and LinAcs has been found to be related to levels of expenditure.[7] In fact supply per million population of this technology is slightly higher in England than Scotland, but is below OECD average in both countries. This indicates that supply patterns in Scotland are an exception to the rule.

We can confidently say that Scotland benefits from more acute hospital beds, more doctors and more nurses per capita. This is as we would expect given extra expenditure in Scotland. International evidence suggests that the number of doctors per head can affect medical outcomes. For example, infant and maternal mortality are significantly reduced when the number of physicians increases.[8] It has also been found that avoidable mortality, when medical intervention is capable of having an impact, also improves with the number of doctors.[9] Here Scotland appears to be an exception to the general rule.

Scottish healthcare provision is more integrated than that in England, while, in terms of scale and geography, the Scottish NHS is arguably more centralised. This may account for some of the differences in outcomes between England and Scotland, but our findings only allow us to speculate on this; remembering the predominantly scathing commentary on the recent comparison of the NHS in England with Kaiser Permanente,[10] which warns us against comparing apples with oranges without a note of caution.[11]

## On Population and Environmental Inputs

A wealth of international evidence suggests that environmental factors (genetic, physical, economic and social) are the most important determinants of a population's health. It is unfortunate that these elements largely lie outside the scope of this paper. Nevertheless, looking at exercise patterns, fat, fruit and vegetable, alcohol, and tobacco consumption, it is clear overall, that the Scots lead somewhat less healthy lifestyles than the English, though of course there are important variations between sexes and different age-groups. Leon and his team note two worrying differences among young females: 'Levels of hypertension were greater in Scottish females aged 45-64 and levels of overweight and obesity were significantly higher in young Scottish females (16-24) than in English females in the same age-groups'.[12] And again, the geographical variation within both Scotland and England should be emphasised. Indeed there are regions in England, which have poorer environmental inputs than many parts of Scotland.

## The 'Scottish Effect'[13]

The role of socio-economic deprivation has been at the centre of much analysis of Scotland's health outcomes.[14] Carstairs' work, which examines the extent to which differences in deprivation levels between Scotland, England and Wales, explain differences in mortality, being most well-known[15] Carstairs showed that a larger proportion of the Scottish population lives in the most deprived areas.[16] However, more recent research qualifies this 'Scottish Effect'. David Leon et al. of LSHTM, do not rule it out but sound a note of caution. Using findings from a recent ONS publication,[17] they argue that: 'Perhaps the most striking thing about these analyses is the fact that the absolute differences in mortality between Scotland and England are small in the least deprived and largest in the most deprived category. This applies to all causes, lung cancer and coronary heart disease [which] undermines the notion of a fixed "Scottish effect" that applies equally to everyone in Scotland.'[18] Leon *et al.* consider that the 'Scottish Effect' should be recognised for what it is: 'simply a description that deprivation as measured by the Carstairs-Morris index does not explain differences in mortality between constituent parts of the UK'.[19] Scotland does have an unfavourable distribution of deprivation in its population,[20] and the Public Health Institute for Scotland (PHIS) also suggests that, if we look at premature mortality for those under 65, deprivation explains c. 60 per cent of the excess, though not the other 40 per cent.[21] So how do we explain the remaining excess? Referring back to our inputs/outputs model, perhaps education, environment and so forth play a role, as do poor diet and above average exposure to tobacco and alcohol, but we should not underestimate the importance of the health system itself.

### On Health Outcomes

Overall, and contrary to common belief, though health funding has been higher in Scotland for many years, health outcomes are not uniformly worse in Scotland than in England. Perhaps commentators who take that line are simply examining life expectancy—a measure which is thought by many to indicate little about a health system's performance. Nevertheless, the hypothesis we examined is supported by the evidence, albeit with some qualification. Outcomes in Scotland are generally speaking worse, but some are equal or slightly better than those in England. Whether this is because of fundamental health system flaws, genetics or unhealthy lifestyles we cannot really say. However, we can pose legitimate questions about causality. If we take those international studies by the OECD and others which looked at funding, resource levels and outcomes, Scotland seems to swim against the tide. And it is important to recall that this has not always been the case. As Leon *et al.* write: 'Scotland has not always performed so poorly. In the first half of the twentieth century life expectancy was actually higher for both men and women than in a number of Western European countries, such as France, Spain and Italy. In the middle of the twentieth century, however, things started to go wrong.'[22] Although life expectancy has increased in Scotland (and England), rates of increase in other countries were faster.

Health outcomes in Scotland are most notably worsened by the very high mortality rates among working-age adults.[23] But Leon *et al.* note again that high cancer and cardiovascular disease mortality, especially among women, is 'not an exclusively Scottish phenomenon. While Scotland may have fared worse, it exhibits a pattern that is similar to that seen in other parts of the British Isles.'[24] In an international context we can confidently state that both England and Scotland remain weak performers; the latest publication of the OECD's health data (2003) again shows the poor quality of UK healthcare compared to other countries.[25] The statistics show that victims of heart disease, stroke or cancer in Britain die early and unnecessarily compared with most other western countries. So will simply spending more on health care in England (albeit alongside the introduction of some supply-side flexibility) lead to health outcomes like those in Switzerland or France?

## Discussion

Do these findings suggest that the NHS (in England and perhaps even more so Scotland) suffers from a systemic flaw that can only be overcome by radical change? Have other systems proved better able to avoid rationing by keeping the resources available for treatment in balance with medical demand?[26] Are there other systems that are better at turning resource inputs into outputs and outcomes, notwithstanding deprivation? Our main aim was to explore the hypothesis that increasing healthcare expenditure in England may not yield improvements in patient care sufficient to raise England to the standards found in countries such as Switzerland and France. This hypothesis is supported, albeit with the 'health-input' related caveats mentioned above, by our collated evidence; Scotland's increased resources have not given rise to a step change in health outcomes—though some may argue that outcomes would be much worse without its extra funding.

One reason for this performance deficit in England and Scotland may be that the UK government has a near monopoly over the funding and provision of health care. After decades of political control, English healthcare spending is comparatively low, but is set to match the EU average over the next few years. But there is no reason to suppose that current increases in funding will continue in the long term, while political control remains so strong. Even if we could guarantee sustained increase in public funding, it could be said that, in relation to a health system, expenditure per head is not the most important factor in determining health outcomes. Scotland arguably teaches us that.

In 2002, the OECD ARD team also published findings of a study which had examined elements of health systems that influence CHD treatment (see Table 6.1). They found that tax-funded systems (Canada, Denmark, Norway and the UK) were most likely to restrict the number of specialist units (revascularisation facilities), and would also have the lowest number of such facilities. Meanwhile, the artificial restriction of such facilities was weakest in social insurance countries (Belgium, Switzerland and Germany).[27]

The relationship between utilisation and demand was examined by the OECD ARD team.[28] They found the level of CHD to be a reasonably reliable indicator of demand for PTCA and CABG. Table 6.1 below shows that countries with high rates of CHD like Germany and the US have correspondingly high revascularisation rates. The converse applies for Italy. However, the relationship is more complex as Belgium and Switzerland, countries with low levels of CHD, have higher revascularisation rates than most countries, including the UK and Hungary, which have much higher levels of CHD. The OECD team concluded that the main contributory factor to high levels of use in social-insurance based Belgium and Switzerland is the lower influence of supply-side constraints.[29] In their discussion, and without inferring what would be considered the optimal utilisation rate for a given level of CHD, they conclude that there is a weak relationship between level of CHD and utilisation rates for revascularisation procedures. Deviating significantly from the trend line, insurance-based US, Belgium and Germany perform more revascularisations than one would expect, while tax-funded Italy, Spain, the UK and Denmark perform fewer. Given their relatively high levels of CHD, Denmark and the UK perform particularly low numbers of revascularisations.

Both CABG and PTCA treatment require special equipment. The ARD team found that the number of facilities equipped to perform the procedures is correlated with the utilisation levels of those procedures. The US performs the largest number of CABG procedures and has the highest number of cardiac surgery facilities per 100,000 population.[30] This relationship is stronger for PTCA. The variation in the supply of specialist facilities can be explained by the imposition of supply-side constraints. This regulation tends to be greater in countries reliant on general taxation than in social insurance countries.[31] Consequently, none of the countries with strong constraints (Canada, Denmark, Norway, the UK) had high utilisation for revascularisation procedures. The converse applies in Belgium, Switzerland, Germany and the US, where limited regulation was associated with high rates of utilisation (see Table 6.1).

Provider payment methods appear to have similar effect to the regulatory régime; countries where fee-for-service is the main payment method for hospitals and physicians, have high levels of revascularisation.[32] In the UK, with global budgets for hospitals and physicians paid by salary, revascularisation rates are among the lowest.[33] If utilisation rates and levels of CHD are plotted on a chart, it is striking that countries below the trend line all pay physicians on a salary basis—and all are tax-financed countries. Before drawing firm conclusions from this OECD evidence, we should caution readers that an earlier Civitas research project comparing healthcare outcomes and health funding and provision systems in nine countries failed to find conclusive evidence of a link between the health system and health outcomes.[34]

One of the common arguments in favour of tax funding is based on the myth that taxation is the most efficient means to pay for health care. This is simply wrong. Any system can be inefficient.[35] Although OECD member countries with systems funded through social insurance have higher average total expenditure on health (a potential indicator of wasteful spending), tax funding can be as inefficiently spent as any other type of funding. Perhaps Scotland demonstrates this. The Netherlands and Germany illustrate that cost control can be effective in insurance systems.[36] It is the systems and incentives under which providers, payers and patients operate that are important when considering technical efficiency. In 2002, Mossialos and Dixon hypothesised that typically higher spending in social insurance systems could be owing to greater transparency, less political interference, greater connection between contributions and benefits, and the existence of single or multiple insurers.[37] Another NHS myth has been highlighted by this study: the myth that health care in the UK is based on need, not ability to pay.

### Ensuring Access for the Poor

In reality, access to care in the UK is influenced by age, gender, education, race, class and wealth. We have multi-tier systems in both England and Scotland, though private care is more common in England. Almost all developed countries claim that their citizens have access to healthcare on the basis of need not ability to pay.[38] To continue to claim or suggest that the NHS is different in this respect is dishonest. Many countries can make this claim with more authority than the UK. In a speech to the Fabian Society, Tony Blair underlined again that the health system in

Britain is now clearly a two multi-tier service with the rich getting treatment denied to the poor—precisely the problem that the NHS was meant to address.[39] It is paradoxical that the chief reason for widespread public support of the NHS is its promise to care for everyone, regardless of income.

Despite the growing multi-tier health service in Britain, the NHS does in principle offer equal treatment to rich and poor alike. It is axiomatic that those on low incomes should have access to high quality medical services, and that no one should be denied access to essential treatment because they cannot afford it. While this is meant to be one of the strengths of the NHS, it is my contention that social insurance systems such as those in Switzerland, France, and Germany achieve this far better, ensuring their poor get better treatment than they do in the UK. Certain system features or characteristics associated with social insurance and tax-based systems are presented in Table 6.2.

## Table 6.1
### Level of CHD, supply constraints and utilisation of revascularisations

| | Utilisation of revascularisation procedures | | |
|---|---|---|---|
| | *High* | *Medium* | *Low* |
| High level of CHD | AUS, GER, USA | CAN, DNK, FIN, NOR, SWE | HUN, UK |
| Low level of CHD | BEL, CH | ESP, GRC, JPN, KO | ITA |
| *SUPPLY CONSTRAINTS* | | | |
| REGULATION OF FACILITIES | Utilisation of revascularisation procedures | | |
| | *High* | *Medium* | *Low* |
| *Strong constraint* | AUS | CAN, DNK, NOR | UK |
| *Medium constraint* | | FIN, GRC, ITA, SWE | HUN |
| *Low constraint* | BEL,CH, GER, USA | ESP, JPN, KOR | |
| HOSPITAL PAYMENT METHODS | *High* | *Medium* | *Low* |
| *Global budgets* | | CAN, DNK, ESP, GRC, NOR, SWE | UK |
| *Mixed financing* | AUS, USA | FIN | HUN, ITA |
| *Fee-for-service* | BEL, CH, GER | JPN, KOR | |
| PHYS PAYMENT METHODS | *High* | *Medium* | *Low* |
| *Salaried* | AUS, GER | DNK, ESP, FIN, JPN, NOR, SWE | HUN, ITA, UK |
| *Mixed remuneration* | AUS, GER | CAN, GRC | |
| *Fee-for-service* | BEL, CH, USA | KOR | |

Key: AUS–Australia; CH–Switzerland; ESP–Spain; GRC–Greece
*Source:* adapted from OECD, ARD Team study findings, 2002

## Table 6.2
### System features / characteristics associated with social insurance and tax-based systems

| System features/ characteristics | Other comments | Social Insurance systems | Tax-based systems |
|---|---|---|---|
| Supply side constraints | | Low | High |
| Access to radiation therapy | | Easier | Serious delays |
| No of revascularisation procedures performed | | Higher than expected | Lower than expected |
| Spending level | | Higher | Low |
| Financial transparency | Between contributions and benefits | Higher, degree depends on collection mechanism | Low, though higher in some decentralised systems |
| Number of specialist stroke units (SSUs) | SSUs were adopted earlier and faster in public integrated systems (Scandinavia) | No clear trend | No clear trend<br>Low in the UK |
| Rate of mammography | Tends to be higher in public integrated systems | No clear trend | No clear trend<br>UK among lower use group |
| No. of mammography machines | | Higher, if few constraints on technology diffusion | Tend to be lower in countries with explicit constraints on technology diffusion |
| Public health priorities | | Weak tendency to be treatment orientated. Some conflict of interest | Weak tendency to be prevention orientated |
| Hospital payment constraints | | Weaker (except NL) | Strong |
| Payment systems | | Flexible (fee-for-service, DRGs) | Fixed (global budgets) |

*Source:* based on Civitas research and the findings of the OECD Ageing Related Disease Study Programme

# Commentary

# Kevin Woods

The observed trend for healthcare expenditures to grow more rapidly than the GDP of individual countries poses substantial dilemmas for citizens and governments alike.[1] Both want better health and health care, and they want also to maximize the efficiency of acquiring them. Wherever we look in the developed economies, a central problem posed by the health sector is how to reconcile these two competing forces. How can levels of provision be improved whilst costs are contained? Compared with many other countries the UK has historically had effective control of public healthcare expenditures, but quality shortcomings have become matters of public concern. However, comparative studies of health care have paid most attention to policy or system inputs (levels of health spending, especially from public sources, numbers of physicians and beds per capita). The policy problem now, and the challenge to comparative research, is not what costs least, but what works best. In this way, the nascent interest in and use of benchmarking in health care reflects and shapes a new attention to outputs and outcomes (health indicators, patient satisfaction). It is an interest that goes beyond health policy and is relevant to many other aspects of government activity.[2] Whilst many of the determinants of health are acknowledged to lie outside the healthcare delivery system,[3] there is increasing evidence that the quality of health care and access to it do have important contributions to make to

This commentary draws on an earlier unpublished paper prepared in conjunction with Helen Alexander, University of Glasgow, John Bullivant, Health & Social Care Quality Centre Wales, Neil Craig, University of Glasgow, and Richard Freeman, University of Edinburgh and is used with their agreement.

population health, both in terms of life expectancy and quality of life.[4] In short, the organisation of health care matters and healthcare systems vary in their ability to convert the human and financial resources at their disposal into treated patients and improved health.

## Using Cross-National Information in Domestic Policy

Governments pursue these interests in an increasingly international context. Health and health care are themselves increasingly influenced by factors outside the direct control of individual governments.[5] Rapidly evolving information technologies and improved communications of all kinds speed the transfer of ideas, technologies, information, patients, and healthcare professionals from one healthcare system to another.

Part of this exchange is a growth in the availability of information on the comparative performance of individual health systems. This, of course, is not entirely new. There are existing sources of comparative data (e.g. the OECD datasets and the National Audit Office compendium)[6] and the comparative analysis of health policy and health politics is an established academic endeavour.[7] What is new is an increasing tendency for citizens and governments to publicly justify their demands and their policies by reference to performance in other healthcare systems.[8] The academic, professional and technical debate is beginning to be supplemented by public discourse on these matters as a driver of political responses and, consequently, health policy. The Prime Minister's commitment to increase health spending to the European average is a case in point, reflecting the growth in public awareness (fuelled by professional lobbies) of the difference between the proportions of UK GDP spent on health care compared with other countries in the European Union. The publication of the WHO World Health Report[9] took these analyses on to the pages of national newspapers, and recent decisions by the European Court of Justice[10] have ushered in the prospect of cross-border movement of patients to take advantage of 'better services' elsewhere, and a European healthcare policy.[11]

These trends are not limited to the comparison of nation states. There is a growing public interest in the performance of regional health systems within countries that are extending the powers of various forms of regional government e.g. in Italy and Spain. Within the UK, as post-devolution health policy in each of its countries acquires an increasingly distinctive character, there is a growing interest in the comparison of the resources, the policy and the performance of each healthcare system.[12]

## Problems of Measurement

Common to both sets of circumstances—intra- and inter-national—are serious conceptual, methodological and technical problems of comparative health system performance measurement to be overcome. Traditionally, analysis has been dominated by a focus on high-level policy, on resource inputs (e.g. spending or doctors per capita), access (e.g. waiting lists and times), and high-level measures of outcome in the form of life expectancy and mortality rates. This reflects the inherent difficulties of measuring health-care quality and health outcomes in individual health systems. The availability and comparability of data across countries are limited, not least because different countries define health care as a whole, and categories of health care such as hospital services or primary care, in different ways. There are also conceptual problems in drawing inferences about micro-economic relationships between healthcare inputs and health outcomes from aggregate data on expenditure and population health.[13] Policy change typically involves choices at the margin in levels of expenditure or ways of organising health care, the impact of which cannot be reliably inferred from comparisons of aggregate data on historical patterns of expenditure or ways of delivering health care.[14]

Whilst there have been important conceptual and technical developments in the measurement of performance in individual health systems (e.g. each of the UK countries is continuing to develop its own performance assessment framework)[15] it is especially difficult to construct meaningful indicators for the purpose of comparison.[16] There has also been limited systematic incorporation (in the UK at least) of these comparative assessments into the process of policy development through opportunities for policy learning and knowledge transfer.[17]

## Problems of Policy Making

As statistical benchmarking of health system performance develops, it is also important to consider what part it plays (or might play) in health decision-making. It might contribute to the identification of policy problems (to agenda-setting) or of solutions to existing problems (policy formulation). Its function may be superficial and symbolic, legitimating action taken for other reasons, or it may become a source of substantive policy learning. It presents both risks and benefits. The risk is that it inculcates or revives a sense that there might be 'one best way' of delivering health and health care, even though systems of providing and paying for health care are highly complex arrangements deeply embedded in local circumstance. In conditions where uncertainty is high and legitimacy is decreasing, there is some security in doing what others (seem to) do. That is to say that where there are strong tendencies to isomorphism,[18] benchmarking may merely add to normative pressures on governments. Arguably, the consensus that grew through the 1990s in favour of health systems based on forms of social insurance incorporating market-style incentives[19] is an example. On the other hand, benchmarking might serve to heighten self-awareness, reinvigorating discussion of the aims of health policy and the best means of achieving them, informed (even if only indirectly or by imputation) by practice elsewhere.

In the UK context, as patterns of post-devolution health policy begin to be formed, the use of benchmarking raises some specific concerns. Devolution was meant to allow, if not promote, diversity. But it has entailed (more or less by definition) the creation of smaller administrative units, in some ways newly autonomous, in some ways newly vulnerable. So benchmarking of health system performance might

cut either way, or even both ways. But because benchmarking and devolution are both emergent processes, ideas
whose implementation is still in train, there is an important
research agenda that presents a real prospect of shaping
them. The following issues suggest themselves for further
enquiry.

*Performance Measurement and Policy*

- What impact does comparative performance assessment
  have on decision-making and policy development? What
  evidence is there of the link between the expansion in
  performance assessment and policy change? How do
  policy makers utilize analyses of comparative performance in the process of evaluating policy alternatives?

*Diagnostic Indicators*

- Is it possible to define a small number of, or composite,
  'diagnostic' indicators of service and/or clinical quality as
  proxies for the wider array of possible indicators? How
  would individual indicators be weighted in such an
  index? Is it possible to build a 'balanced scorecard' or a
  'maturity matrix' of health systems performance in the
  UK that enables UK health system performance to be
  compared and assessed over time?[20]

*Input / output Relationships*

- What is the nature of the relationship between indicators
  of resource input and indicators of health outcome? What
  can be inferred, for example, about the performance of
  health systems from comparisons of expenditure, real
  resources and population health,[21] given the doubts
  expressed by many authors about the contribution made
  by health services to a country's level of morbidity and
  mortality? Is it possible to develop robust statistical
  models of such relationships that enable resource needs
  to be estimated in individual health systems now and in
  the future?[22]

*Improving Performance by Measuring Performance*

- Does the measurement of health system performance
  improve performance? Do healthcare organisations use

indicators of relative performance to change individual and organisational behaviour in order to secure higher levels of performance? What techniques and tools can help link performance assessment and performance? What are the incentives to act on performance data?[23]

## Benchmarking Performance

- How can 'benchmarks' of health system performance be set? This is analogous to the problem of target setting; how difficult should it be to be hit the target? Does the setting of benchmarks and targets create perverse incentives that distort performance?[24] Is the publication of performance against benchmarks a 'carrot' or 'stick'?

## Political Levels and Measurement

- Are intra-system differences in performance greater than inter-system differences in performance? How do 'sub-national' health systems perform in comparison to similar systems in other places (e.g. deprived urban areas)?

## Patient Assessments of Performance

- Can patient-defined views of quality be built into comparative assessments of system performance? Do current policy directives to involve patients and the public in decisions about health systems need to be based on a sounder knowledge base?[25] Can emerging techniques for capturing patients' views within any one health system[26] be extended to indicate aspects of best practice for comparisons across systems?[27] How should information about health systems performance be presented to the public?[28]

## Knowledge Transfer and Policy Learning

- How is learning and knowledge about health system performance measurement transferred between health systems? Can the link between comparative analysis and learning be improved? How can we avoid 'foreign' evidence falling victim to the perception of 'domestic' policy makers and instead make greater use of evidence and evaluation?[29]

These are all complex and contentious questions. They pose many difficult methodological problems. So where can we start?

## Disseminating Learning: Developing a Policy Dialogue

In the post-devolution UK, assembling the available (incomplete, hard to interpret) data and subjecting it to critical scrutiny and debate is an obvious place to begin. Integral to this approach should be an attempt to link the research endeavour with the world of policy practice and its practitioners as well as producing papers for academic journals and conferences. This is to ensure that the learning is disseminated effectively to decision makers in health systems. There are two other reasons for doing so which derive from problems encountered in cross-national research in social and public policy.[30] They often appear incidental to more theoretical and technical aspects of research design, but solving them may well be essential to a project's success. They are equally relevant in the post-devolution UK.

The first is that of problem definition: comparative research struggles to define its object as other than either an abstract, theory-derived, ideal type or as some lowest common denominator which invariably privileges one set of meanings over others; the concept of 'performance' is no exception to this. The best comparative work takes what is being researched as a differentiated set, sensitive to the variety of ways in which some phenomenon is constructed and configured in different contexts.

The second problem is that of 'relevance', which entails producing knowledge for as well as of policy, and may well include meeting sponsors' demands for the involvement of research users. This is an issue that cross-national projects share with policy-related research of all kinds, but the prior 'problem of problem definition' tends to make it seem even more intractable.

One way forward is to use the idea of the 'policy seminar' employed to address the issues of problem definition and policy relevance in a recent project on cross-national learning in health care.[31] It describes how policy seminars are used to explore the different ways in which issues present in different national contexts, as well as to foster the collaboration of the policy makers identified as its principal potential users. It offers a more efficient and effective way of doing what the focused interview[32] does across national settings. In working with policy elites, it serves also to shift the dynamic between research provider and research user.

### Scotland vs England

In assembling a wealth of data on health and health care in Scotland and England, Civitas has provided an accessible source of raw material for such debate. Imperfect it may be, and open to different interpretations it certainly is, but it offers a useful starting point for careful and critical scrutiny of how two healthcare systems use the resources at their disposal. The numerous endnotes that accompany the data in the paper illustrate the risks of preparing such a paper, in particular just how difficult it is to compare like with like. A predictable (and legitimate) debate about the adequacy of the data, the need for adjustments for this and that, can be anticipated.

Recent studies comparing the performance of the NHS and the American Health Maintenance Organisation, Kaiser Permanente[33] and the costs of healthcare administration in the USA and Canada[34] are excellent examples. The former study has unleashed a huge correspondence in the pages of the *BMJ* as the data and methods are critically examined. This is welcome for two reasons; first it ensures that the quality of the data and the analysis will improve and second because it focuses attention on important differences in health system performance, data limitations notwithstanding. Even so there remain difficult questions about the nature of the relationships within each data set and questions of causality. If the Civitas paper can achieve the same productive, critical engagement as opposed to a rush to defend one system or the other through a common condemnation of the data, it will have made a useful contribution.

One issue that is likely to arise in such discussion is the impact of social deprivation on the Scottish health data. It is beyond doubt that there is a concentration of deprivation in Scotland (notably in the Glasgow city region), which has an adverse effect on health status. This must be remembered when examining the data, but two important points need to be made in the light of recent research that has examined Scotland's health in the context of other European nations.[35] Firstly, not all aspects of Scotland's health record are bad; health in the younger age-groups compares well with others; and viewed historically there is nothing inevitable about Scotland's current situation since in previous decades Scotland's position in the European league table of health has been better. Secondly, the careful analysis of the Public Health Institute for Scotland[36] has shown that, when Scotland is compared with England, the extent of social deprivation in Scotland explains 40 per cent of the excess of all age mortality, and 60 per cent of the observed excess of premature mortality, but the balance is due to other factors, sparking a quest for the answer to the question posed by PHIS of whether there is a particular 'Scottish effect' at work? In view of the increasing evidence of the contribution of modern health care to the length and quality of life, it would be a mistake not to consider carefully, alongside other possible factors, the organisation of healthcare delivery as a contributor to health outcomes.

Where many will part company with the current study is its argument that the transformation of the NHS into a social insurance system would bring improved responsiveness and better health outcomes. In a keynote speech to an OECD conference devoted to the measurement of health system performance, David Naylor reminded his audience of health ministers and leading policy makers that:

> As different countries have gone down different [reform] routes, a hard reality has emerged: there are no 'magic bullets' to be had in healthcare reform. One conclusion—which may be taken as depressing, liberating, or a bit of both—appears to be that improvements in health care are not contingent on the drafting

of grand blueprints or the ability of politicians and public servants to pull big policy levers. Healthcare improvement starts from the ground up. It requires tenacious work to understand what does and does not work in real life and the engagement of countless providers [clinicians] and patients, institutions and communities. Similarly, most policy movement seems to be incremental, driven by experience and evidence, rather than theory or ideology.[37]

From this perspective, a key question is whether the changes advocated by Civitas, even if they were politically feasible, would produce the desired effects?

# Bibliography

Adab, P., Rouse, A., 'Is population coronary heart disease risk screening justified? A discussion of the National Service Framework for coronary heart disease (Standard 4)', *British Journal of General Practice*, October 2001: 834-837.

Adams, J. and Robinson, P. (eds), *Devolution in Practice: public policy differences within the UK*, IPPR, 2002.

Arrow, K., 'Uncertainty and the welfare economics of medical care', *The American Economic Review*, Vol. 53, No. 5, 1963.

Atkinson, A., 'Income Inequality in the UK', *Health Economics* 1999; 8: 283-8.

Audit Commission and CHI, *NHS Cancer Care in England and Wales*, TSO, 2001.

Bechhofer, F. and Paterson, L,. *Principles of Research Design in the Social Sciences,* London: Routledge, 2000.

Bell, D. and Christie, A., 'The Barnett Formula: Nobody's Child?', in Trench, A. (ed.), *The State of the Nations 2001*, Exeter: Imprint Academic. 2001.

Berrino, F., Capocaccia, R., Esteve, J., Gatta, G., Hakulinen, T., Micheli, A., Sant, M., and Verdecchia, A. (eds), *Survival of Cancer patients in Europe: the EUROCARE-2 Study,* IARC Scientific Publications, No. 151, World Health Organisation, International Agency for Research on Cancer, European Commission, Lyon, 1999.

BMA Health Policy & Economic Research Unit, *Healthcare Funding Review,* British Medical Association, 2001.

Blamey, A., Hanlon, P., Judge, K. and Murie, J. (eds), *Health Inequalities in the New Scotland,* PHIS, 2002.

Block, P., Weber, H. and Kearney, P., 'Manpower in cardiology II in Western and Central Europe (1997-2000)', *European Heart Journal,* February 2003, 22; 4: 299-310.

Bodenheimer, T. and Grumbach, K., 'Financing universal health insurance: taxes, premiums and the lessons of social insurance', *Journal of Health Politics, Policy and Law,* Vol. 17, No. 3, 1992, pp. 439-462.

Bolderson, H., Mabbett, D.,Hudson, J., Rowe, M. and Spicker, P., *Delivering Social Security: A Cross-National Study*, Report of research carried out by the Department of Government at Brunel University on behalf of the Department of Social Security, London: Stationery Office, 1997.

Bosanquet, N., *Stroke-Reducing the Burden of Disease*, The Stroke Association, 1999.

British Heart Foundation Statistics Database, British Heart Foundation, 2003.

Brown, P., 'UK death rates from breast cancer fall by a third', *British Medical Journal*, 2000; 321:849.

Browne, A. and Young, M., *NHS Reform: Towards Consensus*, Adam Smith Institute, 2002.

Bullivant, J., *Benchmarking for Continuous Improvement in the Public Sector*, Longman, 1994.

Bullivant, J., *Benchmarking for Best Value in the NHS*, London: Financial Times Healthcare, 1998.

Bunker, J., 'The role of medical care in contributing to health improvements within societies', *International Journal of Epidemiology*, (2001) 30, 1260-1263.

Busse, R., *Health Care Systems: Britain and Germany Compared*, Anglo-German Foundation for the Study of Industrial Society, 2002.

Cameron, D. and Dixon J.M., Letters, 'Postcode prescribing is alive and well in Scotland', *British Medical Journal*, 2002; 325:101 (13 July).

Caminada, K. and Goudswaard, K., *International Trends in Income Inequality and Social Policy*, Paper presented to International Social Security Association's Year 2000 International Research Conference on Social Security, Helsinki, 25-27 September 2000.

Cancer Research UK, *About Cancer* (webdoc):
http://www.cancer research uk.org/aboutcancer/?version=1

Carstairs, V. and Morris, R., 'Deprivation: explaining differences in mortality between Scotland, England and Wales', *British Medical Journal*, 1989; 299:886-9.

Carstairs, V. and Morris, R., *Deprivation and Health in Scotland*, Aberdeen: Aberdeen University Press, 1991.

Christie, B., 'Cancer Centre at "breaking point"', *British Medical Journal*, 2001; 328:1148.

Coebergh, J.W.W., Sant, M., Berrino, F., and Verdecchia, A., and the EUROCARE Working Group., 'Survival of Adult Cancer Patients in Europe diagnosed from 1978-1989: The EUROCARE II Study', *European Journal of Cancer*, Vol. 14, No. 14, 1998.

Coleman, M., Babb, P., *et al.*, *Cancer survival trends in England and Wales, 1971-1995: deprivation and NHS Region*, ONS, Studies in Medical and Population Subjects No. 61, London: TSO, 1999.

Commission for Health Improvement/Audit Commission, 'Who gets cancer and their survival', *National Service Framwork Assessments No. 1, NHS Cancer Care in England and Wales*, supporting data No. 1, 2001.

Cookson, J.B., Cancer survival [Letter], *Lancet*, 356(9241):1611.

Coulter, A. and Cleary, P.D., 'Patients Experiences with hospital care in Five Countries', *Health Affairs*, (2001) 20(3) 244-252.

Coxon, I. and McCall, A. (eds), 'Good Hospital Guide', *Sunday Times*, 6 April 2003, p. 9.

CRAG, *Clinical Outcomes Indicators*, Clinical Resource and Audit Group, Scottish Executive, 2002.

Damhuis, R.A.M., Kirkels, W.J. and the EUROCARE Working Group, 'Improvement in survival of patients with cancer of the kidney in Europe', *European Journal of Cancer*, Vol. 14, No. 14, 1998, pp. 2233-2235.

Davey Smith, G., Dorling, D., Mitchell, R. and Shaw M., 'Health inequalities in Britain: continuing increases up to the end of the 20th century' *Journal of Epidemiology and Community Health*, 2002; 56: 434-435.

Daykin, C., *National Insurance Fund Long Term Financial Estimates*, Report by the Government Actuary's Quinquennial Review of the National Insurance Fund, Government Actuary's Department, 1999.

Daykin, C., *Report by the Government Actuary on the Drafts of the Social Security Benefits Up-Rating Order 2002 and the Social Security (Contributions) (Re-Rating and National Insurance Funds payments) Order 2002.* Government Actuary's Department, 2002.

Deacon, S., *Official Report* SW1-5574, 24 July 2000, Edinburgh, Scottish Parliament.

Deaton, A. and Paxson, C., *Mortality, Income, and Income Inequality Over Time in Britain and the United States*, NBER Working Paper No. w8534, National Bureau of Economic Research, 2001.

Department for Environment, Food and Rural Affairs, *National Food Survey 2000*, London: The Stationery Office, 2001.

Department of Health, Chief Medical Officer's Expert Advisory Group on Cancer, *A Policy Framework for Commissioning Cancer Services,* London: Department of Health, 1995.

Department of Health, *A Survey of Radiotherapy Services in England,* DoH, 1999.

Department of Health, *Breast Screening Programme England: Bulletin 2001-02*, February 2003.

Department of Health, *Building on Experience, Breast Screening Programme Annual Review 2002,* NHS, 2002.

Department of Health, *Cervical Screening Programme England: Bulletin 2002/21*, October 2002.

Department of Health, *Delivering Better Heart Services – Progress Report: 2003*, NHS, 2003.

Department of Health, *Departmental Report 2002-2003,* DoH, London, 2000.

Department of Health, *Expenditure Plans 2002-03 to 2003-04*, Departmental Report, 2002.

Department of Health, *Health of the Nation* DoH, HMSO, 1992.

Department of Health, *Health Survey for England 1998*, The Stationery Office, December 1999.

Department of Health, *Medical and Dental Workforce Statistics,* DoH, 2003.

Department of Health, *Saving Lives: Our Healthier Nation,* Cm.4386, London: TSO, July 1999.

Department of Health, *Statistical Press notice – NHS Waiting List Figures*, 30 September 2002, Press release reference: 202/0470, Friday 15 November 2002.

Department of Health, *The NHS Plan*, Department of Health, 2000.

Department of Health, *The NHS Cancer Plan,* DoH, 2000.

Department of Health, *The NHS Plan, Implementation Programme*, Department of Health, 2000.

Department of Health, *The NHS Cancer Plan – Making Progress* DoH, 2001.

Department of Health, *Your Guide to the NHS*, HMSO, 2001.
http://www.nhs.uk/nhsguide/home.htm
(accessed on 19 February 2003).

Department of Health, *Breast Screening Programme England: Bulletin,
2000-01*, Department of Health, 2002.

Department of Health, *Vacancies Survey, 2002*, Department of Health,
2002.
Dewar, S., *Shaping the new NHS: Government and the NHS: Time for a
new relationship?*, King's Fund, Discussion Paper, October, 2003.

DiMaggio, P.J. and Powell, W.W., 'The iron cage revisited: institutional
isomorphism and collective rationality in organizational fields', in Powell,
W.W. and DiMaggio, P.J. (eds), *The New Institutionalism in Organizational
Analysis*, Chicago: University of Chicago Press, 1991.

District Audit Wales, *'Maturity Matrices'*, January 2001.

Dixon, A. and Robinson, R., 'The United Kingdom', in *Health care systems
in eight countries: trends and challenges*, Commissioned by the Health
Trends Review, HM Treasury, Prepared by the European Observatory on
Health Care Systems, 2002.

Dixon, J., *What is the hard evidence on the performance of 'mainstream'
health services serving deprived compared to non-deprived areas in England?*, Report for the Social Exclusion Unit, September 2000.

Dobson, R., 'Proportion of spending on care for older people falls', *British
Medical Journal*, 2002; 325-355.

Dolowitz, D. and Marsh, D., 'Who Learns What from Whom: a review of the
policy transfer literature', *Political Studies* (1996) XLIV (2) 343-357.

Domenighetti, G. and Quaglia, J., 'Comparaisons internationales', in
Kocher, G. and Oggier, W., *Système de santé Suisse 2001/2002*, Concordat
des assureurs-maladie, 2001.

Donaldson, L. J., Kirkup, W., Craig, N. and Parkin, D., 'Lanterns in the
Jungle: Is the NHS Driven by the Wrong Kind of Efficiency?', *Public Health*,
(1994) 108:3-9.

Ebrahim, S. and Redfern, J., *Stroke Care – A Matter of Chance*, A National
Survey of Stroke Services, The Stroke Association, 1999.

Ecob, R. and Davey Smith, G., 'Income and health: what is the nature of the
relationship?', *Social Science & Medicine,* 48, 1999, pp. 693-705.

Emmerson, C. and Frayne, C., *Challenges for the July 2002 Spending Review,*
The Institute for Fiscal Studies, Briefing Note No. 27, 2002.

Entwistle, V.A., 'Supporting and Resourcing Treatment Decision-making: Some Policy Considerations', *Health Expectations* (2000) 3(1) 77-75.

European Court of Justice, *Judgement of the Court, Case C-157/99*, 12 July, 2001.

Evans, M. and Davies, J., 'Understanding policy transfer: a multi-level, multi-disciplinary perspective', *Public Administration* (1999) 77 (2) 361-385.

Faivre, J., Forman, D., Obradovic, M., Sant, M., and the EUROCARE Working Group, 'Survival of patients with primary liver cancer, pancreatic cancer and biliary tract cancer in Europe', *European Journal of Cancer*, Vol. 14, No. 14, 1998, pp. 2184-2190.

Feacham, R.G.A., Neelam, K.S. and White, K.L., 'Getting more for their dollar: a comparison of the NHS with California's Kaiser Permanente', *British Medical Journal*, 2002; 324:135-143.

Forman, D., Gatta, G., Capocaccia, R., Janssen-Heijnen, M.L. and Coebergh J.W., Cancer survival [Comment, Letter], *Lancet*, 357(9255):555, 2001, 17 February.

Forrest, P.A.M., *Breast Cancer Screening, report to Health Ministers of England, Wales, Scotland and Northern Ireland by a working group*, HMSO, 1987.

Freeman, R., *The Politics of Health in Europe*, Manchester University Press, 2000.

Freeman, R., *New Knowledge in New Settings: social learning in the health sector*, European Science Foundation, Standing Committee for the Social Sciences (SCSS), 2001.

Freeman, R. and Woods, K.,'Learning from Devolution: UK Policy Since 1999', *British Journal of Health Care Management*, (2002) Vol 8, (12) 461-466.

Gatta, G., Faivre, J., Capocaccia, R., Ponz de Leon, M., and the EUROCARE Working Group, 'Survival of colorectal cancer patients in Europe during the period 1978-1989', *European Journal of Cancer*, Vol. 14, No. 14, 1998, pp. 2177-2183.

Gatta, G., Lasota, M.B., Verdecchia, A. and the EUROCARE working Group, 'Survival of European Women with gynaecological tumours, during the period 1978-1989', *European Journal of Cancer*, Vol. 14, No. 14, 1998, pp. 2218-2225.

Gatta, G., Capocaccia, R. and Berrino, F., 'Cancer survival differences between European populations: the UK uneasiness', *British Journal of Cancer*, 85(6):785-6, 2001, 14 September.

Gravelle, H. and Sutton, M., 'Income-related inequalities in self-assessed health in Britain: 1979-1995', *Journal of Epidemiology and Community Health*, 2003; 57: 125-129.

Green, D.G. and Caspar, L., *Delay, Denial, Dilution*, Choice in Welfare No. 55, IEA Health and Welfare Unit, 2000.

Green, D. and Irvine, B. (eds), *They've Had a Good Innings: can the NHS cope with an ageing population?*, Civitas, 2003.

Gregor, A., *et al.*, 'Management and survival of patients with lung cancer in Scotland diagnosed in 1995: results of a national population based study', *Thorax* 2001; 56: 212-217.

Gregor, A., 'Foreword', *Cancer in Scotland: Action for Change, National Implementation Plan 2002/03*, 2002.

Grieve, R., *et al.* on behalf of the European BIOMED II European Study of Stroke Care, 'A Comparison of the Costs and Survival of Hospital-admitted Stroke Patients across Europe', *Stroke*, 2001; 32: 1684-1691.

Griffiths, C. and Fitzpatrick, J., *Geographic Variations in Health*, DS No. 16, London: HMSO, 2001.

Grubaugh, S.G. and Santerre, R.E., 'Comparing the Performance of Health Care Systems: An Alternative Approach', *Southern Economic Journal*, (1994) 60, 4, 1030-1042.

Guest, J. and Varney, S., *Alcohol Misuse in Scotland: Trends and Costs*, Catalyst Health Economic Consultants Ltd, Scottish Executive, 2001.

Ham, C., *Health Care Reform: Learning from International Experience*, Buckingham: Open University Press, 1997.

Hanlon, P. *et al.*, *Chasing the Scottish Effect: why Scotland needs a step-change in health if it is to catch up with the rest of Europe*, Public Health Institute of Scotland, 2001.

Heart, 'Fifth report on the provision of services for patients with heart disease', Supplement, *Heart*, 2002; 88 (Suppl III): iii1-iii59.

Hopkins, T.J., 'US cancer mortality may be underestimated', *British Medical Journal*, 2002; 325:182.

HM Treasury, *Public Expenditure Statistical Analyses 2002-2003*, The Stationery Office, 2002.

HPCG, *Consensus Statement*, London: Health Policy Consensus Group, 2002.

HPCG, *Options for Funding*, London: Health Policy Consensus Group, 2003.

HPCG, *Final Report,* London: Health Policy Consensus Group, 2003.

Hughes, M., 'Summary of results from Breast Cancer disease study', in OECD Health ARD Team, *A Disease-Based Comparison of Health Systems: what is best and at what cost?*, OECD, 2003.

Hurst, J., 'Challenges for health systems in Member Countries of the Organisation for Economic Co-operation and Development', *Bulletin of the World Health Organisation,* Vol. 78, No. 6, 2000.

Hurst, J. and Jee-Hughes, M.,'*Performance Measurement and Performance Management in OECD Health Systems*', Labour Market and Social Policy Occasional Papers, No. 47, OECD, January, 2001.

Hurst, J. and Lafortune, G., *Health At a Glance*, OECD Health Policy Unit, Paris: OECD, 2001.

Irvine, B. and Green, D.G., *International Medical Outcomes: How does the UK compare?*, Civitas, 2003.

ISD Scotland, Scottish Cancer Intelligence Unit, *Trends in Cancer Survival in Scotland: 1971-1995*, ISD, Common Services Agency, 2000.

Jacobzone, S., Jee-Hughes, M. and Moise, P., *Medical and Epidemiological Background*, Technical Report, OECD Ageing Related Disease Study, Paris: OECD, 1999.

Jacobzone, S., *The Interplay of Health Policy, Incentives and Regulations in the Treatment of Ageing-related Diseases*, Technical Report, OECD Ageing Related Disease Study, Paris: OECD, 1999.

Janssen-Heijnen, M.L.G., Gatta, G., Forman, D., Capocaccia, R., Coebergh, J.W.W., and the EUROCARE Working Group, 'Variation in survival of patients with lung cancer in Europe', *European Journal of Cancer*, Vol. 14, No. 14, pp. 2191-2196, 1998.

Jee, M. and Or, Z., *Health Outcomes in OECD Countries: A Framework of Health Indicators for Outcome-Orientated Policy Making*, Labour market and social policy – Occasional Papers, No. 36, Paris: OECD, 1999.

Johnston, P. and McDermott, U., *The Principles and Practice of Oncology*, citing Berrino *et al.*, 1995.

Jones T., 'Financing the NHS', in Merray, P. (ed.), *Wellard's NHS handbook 2001/02.*

Kalisch, D., Aman, T. and Buchele, L., *Social and Health policies in OECD countries: a survey of current programmes and recent developments*, Labour market and social policy – Occasional papers, No. 33, Paris: OECD, 1998.

Kanavos, P., *Policy Futures for UK Health: Economy and Finance*, Technical series No. 5, London: The Nuffield Trust, 1999.

Kanavos, P. and Mossialos E., 'International comparisons of healthcare expenditures: what we know and what we do not know?', *Journal of Health Services Research and Policy,* (1999) 4(2), 122-126.

Keaney, M., Lorimer A.R. 'Auditing the implementation of SIGN clinical guidelines' *International Journal of Health Care Quality Assurance*, 9 December 1999, Vol. 12, No. 7, pp. 31-31(1).

Kennedy, B.P., Kawachi I., and Prothrow-Stith D., 'Income distribution and mortality: cross sectional ecological study of the Robin Hood index in the United States', *British Medical Journal*, 1996; 312:20.

Kenway, P., Fuller, S., Rahman, M., Street, C. and Palmer, G., *Monitoring Poverty and Social Exclusion in Scotland*, New Policy Institute and Joseph Rowntree Foundation, 2002.

Klein, R., 'Risks and benefits of comparative studies: notes from another shore', *Milbank Quarterly* (1991) 69 (2) 275-291.

Klein, R., 'Learning from others: shall the last be the first?' *Journal of Health Politics, Policy and Law* (1997) 22 (5) 1267-1278.

Koen, V., *Public Expenditure Reform: The Health Care Sector in the United Kingdom,* Economics Department Working Papers, No. 256, Paris: OECD, 2000.

Laing & Buisson, *Laing's Healthcare Market Review 2002-2003*, London: Laing & Buisson, 2003.

Lampe, F.C., Whincup, P.H., Wannamathee, S.G., Shaper, A.G., Walker, M. and Ebrahim, S., 'The natural history of prevalent ischemic heart disease in middle-aged men', *European Heart Journal* (2000), 21; 1052-1062.

Langhorne, P. *et al.,* of Stroke Unit Trialists' Collaboration, 'Collaborative systematic review of the randomised trials of organised inpatient (stroke unit) care after stroke', *British Medical Journal,* 1997; 314:1151.

Langhorne, P. and Dennis, M., *Stroke Units: an evidence based approach,* BMJ Books, 1998.

Leon, D., Morton, S., Cannegieter, S. and McKee, M., *Understanding the Health of Scotland's Population in an International Context: A review of current approaches, knowledge and recommendations for new research directions*, Part 1, LSHTM, November 2002 (Revised).

Lindley, R.I., Amayo, E.O., Marshall, J., Sandercock, P.A.G., Dennis, M. and Warlow, C.P., 'Hospital Services for patients with acute strokes in the United

Kingdom: The Stroke Association survey of consultant opinion', *Age and Ageing* (1995), 24: 525-532.

Mandelblatt, J.S., Berg, C., Meropol, N., Edge, S., Gold, K., Yi-Ting, H. and Hadley, J., 'Measuring and predicting surgeons' practice styles for breast cancer treatment in older women', *Medical Care*, Vol. 39 (3), pp. 228-242.

Marmor, T.R., Okma, K.G.H., 'Cautionary lessons from the west: what (not) to learn from other countries' experiences in the financing and delivery of health care', in Flora, P., de Jong, P.R., Le Grand, J. and Kim, J-Y. (eds), *The State of Social Welfare, 1997*, International studies on social insurance and retirement, employment, family policy and health care, Aldershot: Ashgate, 1998.

Marshall, M., Shekelle, P., Brook, P. and Leatherman, S., *Dying to Know, Public Release of Information about Quality of Health Care*, Nuffield Trust Series No. 12, Co-published with RAND, 2000.

Mayor, S., 'Review of cancer services shows poor coordination in NHS', *British Medical Journal*, 2001; 323:1383.

Mayor, S., 'UK improves cancer control', *British Medical Journal*, 2003; 326:72.

Merton, R. and Kendall, P., 'The Focused Interview', American *Journal of Sociology* (1946) 51 (6) 541-557.

Melling, P.P., Hatfield, A.C., Muers, M.F., Peake, M.D., Storer, C.J., Round, C.E., Howard, R.A. and Crawford, S.M., 'Lung cancer referral patterns in the former Yorkshire region of the UK', *British Journal of Cancer* 2002; 86: 36-42.

McKee, M. and Figueras, J., 'Strategies for health services', in Detels, R., McEwan, J., Beaglehole, R. and Tanaka, H. (eds), *Oxford Textbook of Public Health*, Oxford: OUP, 2002, pp. 889-909.

McKee, M. and Figueras, J., 'Comparing healthcare systems: how do we know if we can learn from others?', *Journal of Health Services Research and Policy*, (1997) 2(2), 122-125.

McKeown, T., *The Role of Medicine : dream, mirage or nemesis?*, London: Nuffield Provincial Hospitals Trust, 1976.

Morris, C., *The Pocket Guide to NHSScotland 2001/2002*, The NHS Confederation, 2001.

Morris, C., *The Pocket Guide to NHS England 2001/2002*, The NHS Confederation, 2001.

Mossialos, E., Dixon A., Figueras, J. and Kutzin, J. (eds), *Funding Health Care: Options for Europe*, European Observatory on Health Care Systems, Buckingham: Open University Press, 2002.

Mossialos, E. and Le Grand, J., *Health Care and Cost Containment in the European Union*, Aldershot: Ashgate Press, 1999.

Mossialos, E. and McKee, M., 'Is a European Healthcare Policy emerging?', *British Medical Journal*, 2001; 323: 248.

Mossialos, E. and Thomson, S., *Voluntary Health Insurance in the European Union*, European Observatory on Health Care Systems and LSE Health, 2002.

Mulligan, J., Appleby, J. and Harrison, A., 'Measuring the Performance of Health Systems', *British Medical Journal*, 2000; 321:191-192.

National Audit Office, *'Measuring the Performance of Government Departments'*, House of Commons Paper 301, London: The Stationery Office, 14 March 2001.

National Audit Office, *International Health Comparisons*, NAO, 2003.

Navarro, V., 'Assessment of the World Health Report 2000', *Lancet* (2000) 356 (4) 1598-1601.

Naylor, D., Karey, I. and Handa, K., 'Measuring Health System Performance: Problems and Opportunities in an Era of Assessment and Accountability', Paper in 'Measuring up: Improving Health Systems Performance in OECD Countries' *OECD Conference*, Ottawa, 5 November, 2001.

NCEPOD, *Changing the Way we Operate*, Report of the National Confidential Enquiry into Patient Outcome and Death, 2001.

NHS Executive, *The NHS Performance Assessment Framework*, Department of Health, 1999.

NHS Modernisation Board, *The Annual Report (2003) of the NHS Modernisation Board,* March 2003.

NHS Wales, *Improving Health in Wales: A Plan for the NHS and its Partners*, Cardiff: National Assembly for Wales, 2001.

NYCRIS, *Cancer Treatment Policies & their Effects on Survival,* Cancer Outcomes Monitoring, Key Sites Study 2 - Lung Report, Northern and Yorkshire Cancer Registry and Information Service, Leeds, 1999.

OECD, *Health Data: A Comparative Analysis of 33 Countries*, Paris: OECD and CREDES, 2002.

OECD, ARD Team, 'Summary of Results from Ischaemic Heart Disease Study', *What is Best and at What Cost? OECD Study on Cross-National Differences of Ageing Related Diseases*, OECD Working Party on Social Policy, Ageing-Related Diseases, Concluding Workshop, Paris, 20-21 June 2002.

188     ENGLAND VERSUS SCOTLAND

OECD, ARD Team, 'Summary of Results from Breast Cancer Disease Study', *What is Best and at What Cost? OECD Study on Cross-National Differences of Ageing Related Diseases*, OECD Working Party on Social Policy, Ageing-Related Diseases, Concluding Workshop, Paris, 20-21 June 2002.

OECD, ARD Team, 'Summary of Stroke Disease Study' (Draft), *What is Best and at What Cost? OECD Study on Cross-National Differences of Ageing Related Diseases*, DEELSA/ELSWP1/ARD(2002)4. OECD Working Party on Social Policy, Ageing-Related Diseases, Concluding Workshop, Paris, 20-21 June 2002.

OECD, *Health Data: A Comparative Analysis of 33 Countries*, OECD, Paris, 2003.

OECD Health, ARD Team, *A Disease-Based Comparison of Health Systems: what is best and at what cost?*, OECD, Paris, 2003.

Okma, K.G.H., 'Health Care, Health Policies and Health Care Reforms in the Netherlands', *International Publication Series Health, Welfare, and Sport*, No. 7, 2001.

Oliver, A.J., *Risk Adjusting Health Care Resources Allocations*, Office of Health Economics, 1999.

Office for National Statistics, *Living in Britain: Results from the General Household Survey 2000*, London: The Stationery Office, 2001.

Office for National Statistics, *The National Diet and Nutrition Survey: adults aged 19 to 64 years*, ONS, 2002.

Office for National Statistics, *Regional Trends 37*, ONS, 2002.

Or, Z., 'Out-performing or Under-performing: An analysis of health outcomes in France and other OECD countries', *Health and System Science*, Vol. 1,1997, pp. 321-344.

Or, Z., *Exploring the Effects of Health Care on Mortality Across OECD Countries*. Labour market and social policy – Occasional Papers, No. 46, Paris: OECD, 2000.

Or, Z., 'Determinants of health outcomes in industrialised countries: a pooled cross-country, time-series analysis', *OECD Economic Studies*, Vol. 2000/1, No. 30, 2000A.

Parkin, D., 'Comparing health service efficiency across countries', *Oxford Review of Economic Policy*, (1989) 5(1), 75-88.
Parsons, L., *Global Health: A Local Issue*, 2000.
http://www.nuffieldtrust.org. uk/health2/global.intro.doc

Partridge, M., 'Thoracic surgery in a crisis', *British Medical Journal*, Editorial 2002; 324:376-77.

Pell, J., Pell, A.C.H. *et al.*, 'Effect of socio-economic deprivation on waiting time for cardiac surgery: retrospective cohort study', *British Medical Journal*, 2000; 320:15-17.

Petersen, S., Rayner, M. and Press, V., *Coronary Heart Disease Statistics 2000*, London: British Heart Foundation, 2000.

Petersen, S., Rayner, M. and Peto, V., *Coronary Heart Disease Statistics*, London: British Heart Foundation, 2002.

Petersen, S., Rayner, M. and Peto, V., *Coronary Heart Disease Statistics*, London: British Heart Foundation, 2003.

Post, P.N., Damhuis, R.A.M., Van der Meyden, A.P.M., and the EUROCARE Working Group, 'Variation in survival of patients with prostate cancer in Europe since 1978', *European Journal of Cancer*, Vol. 14, No. 14, 1998, pp. 2227-31.

Prior, P., Woodman, C.B. and Collins, S., 'International differences in survival from colon cancer: more effective care versus less complete cancer registration', *British Journal of Surgery*, 85(1):101-4, 1998.

Public Health Institute for Scotland, 2001, *Chasing the Scottish Effect*, PHIS, Clifton House, Glasgow.
www.phis.org.uk

Quinn, M.J., Martinez-Garcia, C., Berrino, F. and the EUROCARE Working Group, 'Variation in survival from breast cancer in Europe by age and country, 1978-1989', *European Journal of Cancer*, Vol. 14, No. 14, pp. 2204-2211, 1998.

Quinn, M., Babb, P., Brock, A., Kirby, L. and Jones, J., *Cancer Trends in England and Wales 1950-1999*, SMPS No. 66, London: ONS, 2001.

Radaelli, C.M., 'Policy transfer in the European Union: institutional isomorphism as a source of legitimacy', *Governance* (2000) 13 (1) 25-44.

Rice, N. and Smith, P., *Approaches to Capitation and Risk Adjustment in Health Care: An International Survey*, Centre for Health Economics, University of York, 1999.

Roberts, M. *et al.*, 'Organisation of services for acute stroke in Scotland – report of the Scottish stroke services audit', *Health Bulletin* 58 (2) March 2000.

Robinson, R. and Dixon, A., United Kingdom, *Health Care Systems in Transition* Copenhagen, European Observatory on Health Care Systems, 1999.

Rodgers, G. B., 'Income and inequality as determinants of mortality: an international cross-section analysis', *International Journal of Epidemiology* 2002; 31:533-538.

Royal College of Physicians, *The National Sentinel Audit of Stroke 1998-99*. Royal College of Physicians of London, July 1999.

Royal College of Physicians, *Summary Report on the National Sentinel Stroke Audit 2001-02*. Royal College of Physicians of London, July 2002.

Royal College of Radiologists, Board of the Faculty of Clinical Oncology, *Medical Manpower and Workload in Clinical Oncology*, London: Royal College of Radiologists, 1991.

Royal College of Radiologists, *Workload, Workforce and Equipment in Departments of Clinical Radiology in Scotland*, London: Royal College of Radiologists, 1999.

Royal College of Radiologists, *Equipment, Workload and Staffing for Radiotherapy in the UK*. London: Royal College of Radiologists, 2000.

Royal College of Radiologists, *Equipment, Workload and Staffing for Radiotherapy in Scotland 1992-1997*, London: Royal college of Radiologists, 2000.

Royal College of Radiologists, *Clinical Radiology: A Workforce in Crisis*. London: Royal College of Radiologists, 2002.

Royal College of Radiologists, The Society of Radiographers, The Institute of Physics and Engineering in Medicine, *UK Radiotherapy Survey, 2002*, A Multidisciplinary Survey of Radiotherapy Services in the UK at 4 June 2002. Available at: http://www.cancernw.org.uk/reports/rtsurvey2002/

Rubin, R. and Mendelson, D., 'A framework for cost sharing policy analysis', in Mattison, N. (ed.), *Sharing the Costs of health: A Multi-county Perspective*, Basle: Pharmaceutical Partners for Better Health, 1995.

Rutstien, D.D. *et al.*, 'Measuring the quality of medical care: A clinical method', *New England Journal of Medicine*, Vol. 294, 1976, pp. 582-88.

Sacks, F.M., Pfeffer, M.A., Moye, L.A., Rouleau, J.L., Rutherford, J.D., Cole, T.G. *et al.*, 'The effect of pravastatin on coronary events after myocardial infarction in patients with average cholesterol levels. Cholesterol and Recurrent Events Trial investigators', *New England Journal Med*, 1996; 335:1001-9.

Sarti, C. *et al.*, 'International Trends in Mortality from Stroke, 1968 to 1994', *Stroke*, 2000; 31: 1588-1601.

SCAN, *Annual Report 2001-2*, South East Scotland Cancer Network, 2002.

Scottish Breast Screening Programme:
http://www.show.scot.nhs.uk/nsd/screening/breast/breast.html

*Scottish Borders Stroke Study*, presented at the European Stroke Conference, Valencia, May 2003.

Scottish Executive, *Cancer in Scotland: Action for Change*. Scottish Executive, The Stationery Office, 2001.

Scottish Executive, *Cancer in Scotland: Action for Change, Annual Report 2002*, Scottish Executive, The Stationery Office, 2002.

Scottish Executive, *Coronary Heart Disease and Stroke Task Force Report*, Scottish Executive Health Department, 2000.

Scottish Executive, *Coronary Heart Disease and Stroke: Strategy for Scotland*, 2002.

Scottish Executive, CMR Monthly Report, *February 1998: Conditions – Stroke*, Information and Statistics Division, NHSScotland, May 1998.

Scottish Executive, *Fair Shares for All: National Review of Resource Allocation*, The Stationery Office, 2000.

Scottish Executive, *National Health Service in Scotland: Annual Report*, 1998-99.

Scottish Executive, *Our National Health: a plan for action, a plan for change*, Scottish Executive Health Department, 2000.

Scottish Executive, *Partnerships for Care*, The Stationery Office, February 2003.

Scottish Executive, *The Scottish Budget 2003-2004*, Annual Expenditure Report of the Scottish Executive, 2003.

Scottish Executive, *The Scottish Health Survey 1998*, Scottish Executive Health Department, November 2000.

Scottish Executive, *Scottish Economic Statistics 2002*, Scottish Executive, 2002.

Scottish Executive, *Workforce Statistics*, Information and Statistics Division NHSScotland. Latest data, 2002 and 2003. http://www.show.scot.nhs.uk/isdonline/NHSiS_resource/Workforce/workforce.htm

Scottish Executive Health Department, Black, R. and Stockton, D. (eds), *Cancer Scenarios: An aid to planning cancer services in Scotland in the next decade*, Edinburgh: The Scottish Executive, 2001.

Scottish Executive Health Department, *New Performance Assessment and Accountability Review Arrangements for NHSScotland*, Edinburgh: Scottish Executive, 2001.

Scottish Executive, NHSScotland, *Scottish Referral Guidelines for Suspected Cancer*, Scottish Executive, 2002.

Scottish Intercollegiate Guidelines Network, *Lipids and the Primary Prevention of Coronary Heart Disease,* SIGN Guidelines No. 40, September 1999.

The Scottish Office, *Designed to Care – Renewing the National Health Service in Scotland,* Cm 3811, The Stationery Office, 1997.

The Scottish Office, *Eating for Health: a Diet Action Plan for Scotland,* The Stationery Office, 1996.

The Scottish Office, *Towards a Healthier Scotland,* The Stationery Office, 1999.

Scottish Parliament Information Centre, *The Barnett Formula,* Research Note RN 00/31, Scottish Parliament Information Centre, May 2000.

SCTS, *National Adult Cardiac Surgical Database Report,* 2000-2001.

Seshamani, M. and Gray, A., 'The impact of ageing on expenditures in the National Health Service', *Age and Ageing,* Vol. 31, No. 4, 2002, pp. 287-94.

Shaw, M., Dorling, D., Gordon, D. and Davey Smith, G., *The Widening Gap: Health Inequalities and policy in Britain,* 1999.

Shepherd, J., Cobbe, S.M., Ford, I., Isles, C.G., Lorimer, A.R., MacFarlane, P.W. *et al.,* 'Prevention of coronary heart disease with pravastatin in men with hypercholesterolemia. West of Scotland Coronary Prevention Study Group', *New England Journal Med.,* 1995; 333: 1301-7.

SIGN, *Lipids and the primary prevention of coronary heart disease,* SIGN Guidelines 40, September 1999.

Sikora, K., 'Rationing cancer care', in Spiers, J., *The Realities of Rationing: 'Priority Setting' in the NHS,* IEA Health and Welfare Unit, Choice in Welfare No. 50. 1999.

Sikora, K., 'Cancer survival in Britain', *British Medical Journal,* 1999, pp. 461-462.

Summerfield, C., Babb, P., (eds), *Social Trends, No. 33.* Office for National Statistics, TSO, 2003.

The Constitution Unit, *Health Policy and Decision Making in a Decentralised System of Government, December 1999—December 2001,* UCL, 2001.

The Stationery Office, *The Social Security Administration Act,* 1992.

The Stroke Association, *Stroke Care - A Matter of Chance,* A National Survey of Stroke Services, The Stroke Association, 1999.

Thomson, S., *Healthcare in Denmark,* Unpublished report commissioned by Civitas, 2002.

Tudor Hart, J., 'Commentary: Three decades of the inverse care law', *British Medical Journal*, 2000, 320: 18-19.

Tunstall-Pedoe, H., Kuulasmaa, K., Mahonen, M., Tolonen, H., Ruokokoski, E. and Amouyel, P., for the WHO MONICA Project (1999), 'Contribution of trends in survival and coronary-event rates to changes in coronary heart disease mortality: 10 year results from 37 WHO MONICA Project populations', *Lancet* 353; 1547-1557.

Van Doorslaer, E. *et al.*, 'Income-related inequalities in health: some international comparisons', *Journal of Health Economics* 1997; 16: 93-112.

Volmink, J.A., Newton, J.N., Hicks, N.R., Sleight, P., Fowler, G.H. and Neil, H.A.W., on behalf of the Oxford Myocardial Infarction Incidence Study Group (1998) 'Coronary event and case fatality rates in an English population: results of the Oxford myocardial infarction incidence study', *Heart* 80; 40-44;

Wade, D., Mant, J. and Winner, S., *Stroke - Healthcare Needs Assessment*, http://hcna.radcliffe-oxford.com/stroke.htm

Wagstaff, A. and Van Doorslaer, E., 'Equity in the delivery of health care: Methods and findings', in Wagstaff, A., Van Doorslaer, E. and Rutten, F., *Equity in the Finance and Delivery of Health Care: An International Perspective*, Oxford: Oxford University Press, 1993.

Wagstaff, A., Van Doorslear, E. *et al.,* 'Equity in the finance of health care: some further international comparisons', *Journal of Health Economics*, Vol. 18, 1999, pp. 263-290.

Wanless, D., *Securing our Future Health: Taking a Long-Term View, Final Report*, London: Her Majesty's Treasury, 2002.

Weir, N. *et al.*, on behalf of the IST Collaborative Group. 'Variations Between Countries in Outcome after Stroke in the International Stroke Trial', *Stroke* 2001; 32: 1370-1377.

Wensing, M. and Grol, R., 'What can patients do to improve health care?', *Health Expectations* (1998) 1(1) 37-49.

Wilkinson, R.G., 'Income distribution and life expectancy' *British Medical Journal*, 1992; 304:165-168.

Wilkinson, R.G., *Unhealthy Societies: the Afflicitons of Inequality*, London, 1996.

Williams, A., 'Science or marketing at WHO? A commentary on 'World Health 2000', *Health Economics*, (2001) 10, 93-100.

Wolfe, C. *et al.*, for the European BIOMED Study of Stroke Care Group. Variations in Case Fatality and Dependency From Stroke in Western and Central Europe, *Stroke 1999*; 30: 350-356.

Wolfe, C. *et al.*, for the European Registries of Stroke (EROS) Collaboration, 'Variations in Stroke Incidence and Survival in Three Areas of Europe', *Stroke* 2000; 31: 2074-2079.

Wolfe, C., McKevitt, C. and Rudd, A. (eds), *Stroke Services – Policy and Practice across Europe*, Radcliffe Medical Press, 2002.

Woodman, C.B., Gibbs, A., Scott, N., Haboubi, N.Y. and Collins, S., 'Are differences in stage at presentation a credible explanation for reported differences in the survival of patients with colorectal cancer in Europe?', *British Journal of Cancer*, 85(6):787-90,14 September 2001.

Woods, K., 'Health Policy and the NHS in the UK 1997-2002', in Adams, J. and Robinson, P. (eds), *Devolution in Practice*, London: The Institute of Public Policy Research (IPPR) and the ESRC, 2002.

Woolhander, S., Campbell, T. and Himmelstein, D.U., 'Costs of Health Care Administration in the United States and Canada', *New England Journal of Medicine*, (2003) 349, 768-775.

World Health Organisation, *Highlights on Health in The United Kingdom*, Draft, Copenhagen, World Health Organisation Regional Office for Europe, 1997.

World Health Organisation, *World Health Report 2000*, Geneva, World Health Organisation, 2000.

World Health Organisation, *European Health For All Database*, Copenhagen, World Health Organisation Regional Office for Europe, 2002.

World Health Organisation, *European Regional Consultation on Health System Performance Assessment*, Regional Office for Europe, Copenhagen, 3-4 September, 2001.

World Health Organisation, The World Health Report, *Reducing Risk Promoting Healthy Life*, World Health Organisation, Geneva, 2002.

Yeun, P. (ed.), *OHE Compendium of Health Statistics*, 14th edn, Office of Health Economics, 2002.

Yngwe, M.A. *et al.*, 'The role of income differences in explaining social inequalities in self-rated health in Sweden and Britain', *Journal of Epidemiology and community Health*, 2001; 55: 556-61.

**Websites:**

British Cardiovascular Intervention Society
www.bcis.org.uk (accessed on 7 February 2004)

Civitas
http://www.civitas.org.uk/pdf/hpcgOutcomes.pdf
(accessed on 7 February 2004)

http://www.civitas.org.uk/pdf/hpcgOutcomesAppendix.pdf
(accessed on 7 February 2004)

The Ecuity Project
www.eur.nl/bmg/ecuity/intro.htm
(accessed on 7 July 2003)

Inland Revenue
www.inlandrevenue.gov.uk/rates/it.htm
(accessed on 13 February 2003)

www.inlandrevenue.gov.uk/education/education4.htm
(accessed on 10 October 2002)

National Audit Office
www.nao.gov.uk
(accessed on 7 February 2004)

BBC
http://news.bbc.co.uk/1/hi/Scotland/2569943.stm
(accessed on 7 March 2003)

National Cancer Services Analysis Team, NHS Executive (North West)
website www.cancernw.org.uk/
(accessed 18 March 2003)

Scottish Health on the Web
http://www.show.scot.nhs.uk/isd/cancer/facts_figures/facts_figures.htm
(accessed on 7 February 2004)

www.show.scot.nhs.uk/isd/primary_care/pservices/pcare_ps_dispensing_
03.htm
(accessed on 7 February 2004)

The Worldbank
www.worldbank.org/data/countryclass/classgroups.htm
(accessed on 7 February 2004)

# *Glossary*

| | |
|---|---|
| AHTs | Acute Hospital Trusts |
| ARD | Ageing Related Disease. The OECD has been carrying out comparative research into diseases of old age (e.g. cancer, stroke and CHD) |
| BCS | Breast-conserving Surgery |
| BMA | British Medical Association |
| BMI | Body Mass Index (a height to weight ratio) |
| BMJ | British Medical Journal |
| BNF | British National Formulary |
| CABG | Coronary Artery Bypass Surgery (a form of revascularisation) |
| CHD | Coronary heart disease |
| CHI | Commission for Health Improvement |
| CSBS | Clinical Standards Board for Scotland |
| CSC | Cancer Services Collaborative |
| CSR | Comprehensive Spending Review |
| CT | (CT-Scan) |
| DoH | Department of Health |
| DRG | Diagnosis Related Groups |
| ECJ | European Court of Justice |
| EUROCARE | Series of comparative cancer survival and treatment studies |
| FMS | Family Medical Services |
| GDP | Gross Domestic Product |
| GMS | General Medical Services |
| HCHS | Hospital and Community Health Services |
| HIPs/ HIMPs | Health Improvement Plans |
| HPCG | Health Policy Consensus Group |
| HTBS | Health Technology Board for Scotland |
| IARC | International Agency for Research on Cancer (of the World Health Organisation) |
| ICD | International Classification of Disease |
| IHD | Ischaemic Heart Disease |
| ISD | Information and Statistics Division (Health statistics in NHSScotland) |

| | |
|---|---|
| LHCCs | Local Health Care Co-operatives |
| LinAc | Linear Accelerator |
| MCNs | Managed Clinical Networks |
| MRI | (MRI-Scan) Magnetic Resonance Imaging |
| NAO | National Audit Office |
| NCEPOD | National Confidential Enquiry into Perioperative Deaths |
| NHS | The National Health Service |
| NHSBSP | NHS Breast Screening Programme |
| NHSQIS | NHS Quality Improvement Scotland |
| NHSScotland | The National Health Service in Scotland |
| NIC's | National Insurance Contributions |
| NICE | National Institute of Clinical Excellence |
| NOSCAN | North of Scotland Cancer Network |
| NRT | Nicotine Replacement Therapy |
| RCAGs | Regional Cancer Advisory Groups |
| NSF | National Service Framework |
| LSHTM | London School of Hygiene and Tropical Medicine |
| OECD | Organisation for Economic Cooperation and Development |
| OHE | Office of Health Economics |
| ONS | Office for National Statistics |
| PCT | Primary Care Trust |
| PET | Positron Emission Tomography |
| PHIS | Public Health Institute for Scotland |
| PMI | Private Medical Insurance |
| PPP | Purchasing Power Parity |
| PTCA | Percutaneous Transluminal Angioplasty (a form of revascularisation) |
| RT after BCS | Breast-Conserving Surgery with Post-Operative Radiation Therapy |
| SBCSP | Scottish Breast Cancer Screening Programme |
| SCAN | South East Scotland Cancer Network |
| SCG | Scottish Cancer Group |
| SCIU | Scottish Cancer Intelligence Unit |
| SEHD | Scottish Executive Health Department |
| SIGN | Scottish Intercollegiate Guidelines Network |

| | |
|---|---|
| TEH | Total Expenditure on Health |
| VAT | Value Added Tax |
| WHO | World Health Organisation |
| WHR | Waist/Hip Ratio |
| WOSCAN | West of Scotland Network |
| WTE | Whole Time Equivalent (as opposed to headcount) |

## Preface

1 HPCG, *Consensus Statement*, Health Policy Consensus Group, 2002.

2 Dewar, S., *Shaping the new NHS: Government and the NHS: Time for a new relationship,* King's Fund, Discussion Paper, October 2003.

3 Dixon, A., Le Grand, J., Henderson, J., Murray, R. and Poteliakhoff, E., *Is the NHS equitable? A review of the evidence*, LSE Health and Social care Discussion Paper Number 11, 2003.

4 HPCG, *Final Report*, Health Policy Consensus Group, 2003.

5 Adapted from: HPCG, *Final Report*, Health Policy Consensus Group, 2003.

6 Note that the little known NHS Information Authority is beginning to provide such information to patients (http://www.nhsia.nhs.uk/def/home.asp).

## Summary

1 Hurst, J., *Challenges for Health Systems in Member Countries of the OECD*, 2000.

2 Or 2000A and Domenighetti and Quaglia 2001. Domenighetti and Quaglia note that infant mortality is correlated with health expenditure. Certain other simple correlations between expenditure and other indicators can be observed: The higher expenditure, the higher the number of beds per 1000, and the greater the length of stays. These two factors do not necessarily affect medical outcomes.

3 The link between expenditure and outcomes is much more significant for women than for men. Or (2000A) considers that this difference in impact on health outcomes may be owing to differences in mortality patterns. Male mortality rates seem less sensitive to medical intervention. 'In most OECD countries, around 30 per cent of the premature mortality for men is a result of "external causes" such as violence, accidents', while for women, cancer is the leading cause of death, accounting for between 20 and 30 per cent, with "external cause" represent only about 16 per cent. Women also benefit from a number of systematic prevention programmes such as screening for cancer, (Or 2000A).

4   In their study of 2001, Domenighetti and Quaglia found the best performing country to be Sweden, which with expenditure of $1,701 per capita, and reveals the best group of indicators— at the top of the scale. The worst performing country from health perspective was found to be the UK—which has a group of indicators at the bottom of the scale. Perhaps observing the diminishing returns, and outlying performers (such as Sweden and the US, the latter was not included in their study), Domenighetti and Quaglia find that avoidable mortality, owing to medical intervention (with or without the inclusion of CHD), is not correlated with health expenditure.

5   Grubaugh and Santerre (1994)

6   Domenighetti and Quaglia 2001, and Or 2000.

7   OECD, ARD team, (2002), 'Summary of Stroke Disease Study', DEELSA/ELSWP1/ARD(2002)4.

8   OECD ARD team, IHD study (2002).

**Introduction**

1   OECD, Health Data, 2003.

2   Dobson, R., 'Proportion of spending on care for older people falls', *BMJ* 2002; 325:355 (17 August).

3   Seshamani and Gray, *Age and Ageing*, 2002, 31 (4): 287-94.

4   Making a connection between a funding system, expenditure, and medical outcomes is fraught with difficulty. The chief problem is that no country has a single system of finance, whereas outcome data are presented for the whole country. We cannot, therefore, be entirely sure whether favourable outcomes are due to the public or private elements of any arrangements. Moreover, competition may be driving performance rather than the funding mechanism and two national systems based on the same funding model may differ in the degree of competition permitted; as is the case in England and Scotland.

5   Model adapted from Busse, R., 2002, pp. 2-3.

6   Busse, R., 2002, pp. 2-3.

7   Theodore Marmor, Professor of Public Policy and Management at the Yale School of Management, and a Visiting Professor in Social Policy at LSE, is famously in the latter camp.

8  See McKee, M. and Figueras J., 'Strategies for health services', in Detels, R., McEwan, J., Beaglehole, R. and Tanaka, H. (eds.), *Oxford Textbook of Public Health*, Oxford: OUP, 2002, pp. 889-909.

9  Leon, D., Morton, S., Cannegieter, S., McKee, M., *Understanding the Health of Scotland's Population in an International Context: A review of current approaches, knowledge and recommendations for new research directions*, Part 1, LSHTM, November 2002 (Revised).

10 Carstairs, V. and Morris, R., 'Deprivation: explaining differences in mortality between Scotland, England and Wales', *BMJ* 1989; 299:886-9. Also see: Carstairs V. and Morris, R., *Deprivation and Health in Scotland*, Aberdeen: Aberdeen University Press, 1991.

11 Leon, *et al.*, 2002, p. 28.

12 Thomson, S., *Healthcare in Denmark*, Report commissioned by Civitas, 2002.

## 1: Healthcare Funding and Expenditure

1  At places in this section of the paper, we use France, Germany, the UK and the USA as comparator countries, in order to put Scotland and England in an international context.

2  OECD, Health Data, 2002.

3  To compare inputs between countries we use Purchasing Power Parities (PPPs) in order to reflect the amount spent, but also healthcare prices in each country (Or, 1997). PPPs equalise the cost of a given 'basket' of goods and services in different countries. Such comparisons merit a cautionary note, as PPP measurement is subject to limitations (OECD, 2002).

4  The Treasury, Public Expenditure Statistical Analyses 2002-2003, Chapter 8. Also see Adams, J., Robinson, P. (eds.), *Devolution in Practice: public policy differences within the UK*, IPPR, 2002, citing, Bell, D. and Christie, A., (2001) 'The Barnett Formula: Nobody's Child?', in Trench, A. (ed.), *The State of the Nations*, Exeter: Imprint Academic, 2001.

5  According to the Office of Health Economics, relative to England, per capita spend on the NHS in 2000/01 was 25 per cent higher in Scotland. Yeun, P. (ed.), *OHE Compendium of Health Statistics*, 14th edn., Office of Health Economics, 2002.

6  Deacon, S., *Official Report* SW1-5574, Edinburgh, Scottish Parliament, 24 July 2000.

7   Scottish Executive, National Health Service in Scotland:
    Annual Report 1998-99. Note that Scottish Executive budget is
    not synonymous with total managed expenditure in Scotland.

8   For an explanation of the workings of the Barnett formula see
    *The Barnett Formula*, Research Note, Scottish Parliament
    Information Centre, May 2000.

9   While the Barnett formula does have some impact on the level
    of healthcare funding in Scotland, it should be seen rather as
    of tangential interest. It must be remembered that a) it only
    applies to funding *increases or decreases* in particular
    departments, and that b) the final funding total is dependant
    on the priorities of the Executive. Thus healthcare funding
    may go up or go down and cannot be easily predicted.

10  *Our National Health: a plan for action, a plan for change*,
    SEHD, 2000, and Scottish Budget 2002-03, pp. 97-98.

11  Wanless, D., *Securing our Future Health: Taking a Long-Term
    View, Final Report*, London: Her Majesty's Treasury, 2002.

12  DoH, NHS expenditure Plans 2002-03; and Emmerson, C. and
    Frayne, C., *Challenges for the July 2002 Spending Review*, The
    Institute for Fiscal Studies, Briefing Note No. 27, 2002.

13  DoH, NHS expenditure Plans 2002-03.

14  Jones, T., 'Financing the NHS', in Merray, P. (ed.), *Wellard's
    NHS handbook 2001/02*.

15  Dixon and Robinson, 2002.

16  In brief, these include varieties of the three main forms of
    public financing (social insurance, local taxation and general
    taxation) and private insurance.

17  OECD researcher Zeynep Or (2000), notes that 'The split
    between the public and private financing of health services
    may influence access to, and use of, medical resources by
    different social groups'. Or (2000A), found evidence of a
    positive impact of public funding on overall mortality and
    morbidity rates.

18  For example, private finance might include private insurance
    (which itself might be substitutive, supplementary or
    complementary), and various user charges. Tax may be direct
    or indirect and may be hypothecated or paid into a general
    pool. Social insurance may be levied in different ways.

19 Department of Health Departmental Report 2002-2003, DoH, London, 2003; Busse, 2002. Also Dixon and Robinson, 2002. These figures are for the UK. Breakdown is different in England and Scotland.

20 Scottish Executive, National Health Service in Scotland: Annual Report 1998-99.

21 www.inlandrevenue.gov.uk/rates/it.htm - accessed on 13 February 2003.

22 www.inlandrevenue.gov.uk/education/education4.htm - accessed on 10 October 2002.

23 The contributions are largely paid to the National Insurance Fund (NIF) and build entitlement to benefits. Contributory benefits include retirement pension, widow's pension, maternity benefit, job seeker's allowance and incapacity benefit. These benefits and their administration are paid for out of the NIF. Many other benefits such as those for disability and support for dependent children are funded from general taxation and are not dependent on contributions.

24 According to the OECD Health Data 2002, public expenditure on health accounted for 14.8 per cent of general government total outlays in 1999. The average expenditure per individual on the NHS was £1,000 in 2002.

25 The Social Security Administration Act 1992, says (s.162 (1)): 'Contributions received by the Inland Revenue shall be paid by them into the National Insurance Fund after deducting from contributions of any class, the appropriate national health service allocation in the case of the contributions of that class.' S162 (5) defines the appropriate NHS allocation: Primary Class 1 contributions—1.05% of contributions; Secondary Class 1—0.9%; Class 1A—0.9%; Class 1B—0.9%; Class 2, 15.5%; Class 3, 15.5%; Class 4, 1.15%. In 1999 combined employee and employer NIC contributions amounted to 22.2% of income. Of that, 1.95% of income was 'allocated' to the NHS. The Treasury insists that the NHS allocation does not simply go into the general tax pool.

26 According to the most recent Government Actuary's Quinquennial Review of the National Insurance Fund. Daykin, C., *National Insurance Fund Long Term Financial Estimates*, Report by the Government Actuary's Quinquennial Review of the National Insurance Fund, Government Actuary's Department, 1999, p. 11.

27 Daykin, C., Report by the Government Actuary on the Drafts of the Social Security Benefits Up-Rating Order 2002 and the Social Security (Contributions) (Re-Rating and National Insurance Funds payments) Order 2002.

28 BMA Health Policy & Economic Research Unit, *Healthcare Funding Review*, British Medical Association, 2001.

29 Yeun, P. (ed.), *OHE Compendium of Health Statistics*, 14th edn., Office of Health Economics, 2002, p. 45.

30 Koen, V., *Public Expenditure Reform: The Health Care Sector in the UK*, Economics Department Working Papers No. 256. OECD, Paris, 2000.

31 Laing and Buisson, *Laing's Healthcare Market Review*, 2002-2003.

32 Laing and Buisson, *Laing's Healthcare Market Review*, 2002-2003.

33 Browne A., and Young M., *NHS Reform: Towards Consensus*, Adam Smith Institute, 2002.

34 Laing and Buisson, *Laing's Healthcare Market Review*, 2002-2003, p. 141.

35 In England and Scotland the following are exempt: children under 16, and young people under 19 in full-time education; those aged 60 and over; expectant mothers; those suffering from certain medical conditions; war pensioners; those receiving certain social security benefits. Note that prescription exemption fraud costs the NHS in Scotland up to £10 million per year.
http://www.show.scot.nhs.uk/isd/primary_care/pservices/pcare_ps_dispensing_03.htm

36 Dixon and Robinson, 2002.

37 NHSScotland and NHS England websites.

38 HSA offers a number of such schemes.

39 Dixon and Robinson, 2002, p. 109.

40 DoH, *NHS Expenditure Plans 2002-03*; and Dixon and Robinson, 2002, p. 109.

41 Comparable data on budget distribution have been difficult to locate. It is likely that expenditure in Scotland of almost £100 million on free care for the elderly, which would represent c. £1 billion *pro rata* in England being spent on health care rather than on social care, would distort the percentages given.

NOTES    **205**

42  Oliver, A.J., *Risk Adjusting Health Care Resources Allocations*, Office of Health Economics, 1999.

43  Rice, N. and Smith P., *Approaches to Capitation and Risk Adjustment in Health Care: An International Survey*, Centre for Health Economics, University of York, 1999.

44  Scottish Health Authorities Revenue Equalisation (SHARE), operated between 1978 and 1998.

45  See World Bank Classifications: http://www.worldbank.org/data/countryclass/classgroups.htm

46  Hurst, 2000.

47  Hurst, 2000; OECD, Health Data, 2002.

48  Hurst, 2000.

49  OECD members countries included in this average: Australia, Austria, Belgium, Canada, Czech Republic, Denmark, Finland, France, Germany, Greece, Hungary, Iceland, Italy, Japan, Luxembourg, New Zealand, Norway, Poland, Portugal, Spain, Sweden, Switzerland, Turkey, United Kingdom, United States. Korea, Mexico, Ireland, Slovakia are omitted.

50  Hurst, 2000.

51  Hurst, 2000.

**2: General Demographic/Environmental Indicators**

1   From Leon, D., Morton, S., Cannegieter, S., McKee, M., *Understanding the Health of Scotland's Population in an International Context: A review of current approaches, knowledge and recommendations for new research directions*, Part 1, LSHTM, November 2002, Revised, p. 8 and p.27.

2   The Scottish NHS Plan states: 'In Scotland our diet, the amount we smoke and drink, and low levels of physical activity are key health determinants.' *Our National Health: A plan for action, a plan for change*, SEHD, 2000.

3   Leon *et al.*, 2002, p. 27.

4   *The National Diet and Nutrition Survey: adults aged 19 to 64 years*, ONS, 2002.

5   Leon, D., Morton, S., Cannegieter, S., McKee, M., *Understanding the Health of Scotland's Population in an International Context: A review of current approaches,*

*knowledge and recommendations for new research directions*,
Part 1, LSHTM, November 2002, (revised), pp. 68-69.

6   BMI (a height: weight ratio) is the most widely used measure
    for overweight or obesity. A BMI of over 25 is classified as
    overweight; a BMI of over 30 is classified as obese; over 40 is
    classified as morbid obesity, a condition recognised as a serious
    illness associated with poor quality of life and co-morbidities
    such as diabetes, cardiovascular disease and hypertension.
    BMI does not differentiate between body weight due to fat and
    body weight due to heaviness, nor does it indicate fat
    distribution.

7   Waist/hip ratio (WHR) is defined as the waist circumference
    divided by hip circumference. WHR is a measure of deposition
    of abdominal fat, i.e. central obesity. There is no consensus as
    to what defines a high WHR and therefore obesity. The
    thresholds here are those chosen by the Joint Health Surveys.

8   Internationally accepted revised guidelines recommend at
    least 30 minutes moderate activity at least five days per week.

9   From Leon *et al.*, *Understanding the Health of Scotland's
    Population in an International Context*, 2002.

10  Hypertension is defined as a systolic blood pressure of greater
    than 140mmHg and/or a diastolic blood pressure of greater
    than 90mmHg. (Leon *et al.*, *Understanding the Health of
    Scotland's Population in an International Context*, 2002.)

11  Leon *et al.*, *Understanding the Health of Scotland's Population
    in an International Context*, 2002.

12  Leon *et al.*, *Understanding the Health of Scotland's Population
    in an International Context*, 2002.

13  The rise in the employment share of white-collar workers (used
    as a proxy for educational and social status), played the
    greatest role in the reduction of premature mortality in most
    countries between 1970 and 1992—more so than increase in
    income (Or, 2000A). Per capita income was the second most
    important factor behind health outcome improvements (Or,
    2000A).

14  Ecob, R. and Davey Smith, G., 'Income and health: what is the
    nature of the relationship?', *Social Science & Medicine*, 48,
    1999, pp. 693-705. Ecob and Davey Smith note that 'a doubling
    of income is associated with a similar effect on health,
    regardless of the point at which this occurs, providing this is

within the central portion (10-90 per cent) of the income distribution'.

15 'Regional studies in several OECD countries have indicated a direct relationship between income inequality and mortality, even after controlling for major risk factors such as alcohol and tobacco consumption' (Or, 2000A – citing Marmot *et al.*, 1984; Helmert and Shea, 1994; Kennedy et al., 1996; Kaplan et al., 1996). Regarding the effect of income inequality on health, see Rodgers, G.B., in *International Journal of Epidemiology* 2002; 31:533-538 (a reprint of his article from 1979). A number of responses to Rodgers' work can be found in the same volume. Also see the work of R. Wilkinson (Wilkinson, R.G., *Unhealthy Societies: the afflicitons of inequality*, London, 1996; and Wilkinson, R.G., 'Income distribution and life expectancy', *BMJ*, 304, 165-168. Rubin, R. and Mendelson, D., 'A framework for cost sharing policy analysis', in Mattison, N. (ed.), *Sharing the Costs of health: A Multi-county Perspective*, Basle: Pharmaceutical Partners for Better Health, 1995.

16 Atkinson, A., 'Income inequality in the UK', *Health Economics*, 1999; 8: 283-8. And Davey Smith G, Dorling, D., Mitchell, R., and Shaw M., 'Health inequalities in Britain: continuing increases up to the end of the 20th century', *Journal of Epidemiology and Community Health*, 2002; 56: 434-435.

17 The Gini Coefficient is a widely used measure of income inequality. It is represented as a percentage or value from 0 to 1, where 0 represents perfect equality and 1 represents perfect inequality. Therefore, the closer the value is to 1 or the higher the percentage, the greater the income inequality.

18 http://www.poverty.org.uk/intro/index.htm; and Kenway, P., Fuller, S., Rahman, M., Street, C. and Palmer, G., *Monitoring Poverty and Social Exclusion in Scotland*, New Policy Institute and Joseph Rowntree Foundation, 2002.

19 Kenway *et al.*, 2002.

20 Gravelle, H. and Sutton, M., 'Income-related inequalities in self-assessed health in Britain: 1979-1995', *Journal of Epidemiology and Community Health*, 2003; 57: 125-129.

21 Van Doorslaer, E. *et al.*, 'Income-related inequalities in health: some international comparisons', *Journal of Health Economics* 1997; 16: 93-112, and Yngwe, M.A. *et al.*, 'The role of income differences in explaining social inequalities in self-rated health in Sweden and Britain', *Journal of Epidemiology and Community Health* 2001; 55: 556-61.

## 3: Healthcare Benefits Package

1   Cited by Dixon, A. and Robinson, R., 2002, p.104.

2   British National Formulary (BNF); and Dixon and Robinson, 2002.

3   Key parts of new legislation are: free personal and nursing care provided by the state—this will represent a 0.2 per cent real-term increase in spending. Personal care is defined as not being help with housing and living costs.

4   Wagstaff, A., Van Doorslaer, E., 'Equity in the delivery of health care: Methods and findings', in Wagstaff, A., Van Doorslaer, E., and Rutten, F., *Equity in the Finance and Delivery of Health Care: An International Perspective*, Oxford: Oxford University Press, 1993. For details of the ECuity project visit the following site: http://www.eur.nl/bmg/ecuity/intro.htm

5   Wagstaff, A., Van Doorslear, E. *et al.*, 'Equity in the finance of health care: some further international comparisons', *Journal of Health Economics*, Vol. 18, 1999, pp. 263-90.

6   Busse, 2002, citing Commission on Taxation and Citizenship, 2000.

7   NICE's remit is to develop authoritative guidance on the clinical and cost effectiveness of treatments. This guidance is intended to provide information on best practice for frontline NHS staff.

8   This obligation falls on the Primary Care Trusts and NHS trusts since they, with the aid of prescribing advisors, now make the decisions on which treatments to fund. Funding decisions were devolved down to them following the changes introduced on 1st April 2002.

9   Keaney, M. and Lorimer, A.R., 'Auditing the implementation of SIGN clinical guidelines', *International Journal of Health Care Quality Assurance*, July 1999, pp. 314-17.

10  See Constitution Unit Quarterly Reports.

11  Cameron, D. and Dixon, J.M., Letters, 'Postcode prescribing is alive and well in Scotland', *BMJ*, 2002; 325:101 (13 July).

## 4: Health System Resources and Organisation

1   There do appear to have been some structural differences between the two systems, such as the inclusion of teaching hospitals within Regional Health Boards in Scotland as

opposed to separate administrations in England and Wales, but most early differences between England and Scotland appear to be matters of degree and emphasis, and certainly appear to be unquantifiable (McTavish, D., 'The NHS: Is Scotland different? A case study of the management of healthcare in the hospital service in the West of Scotland 1947-1987', in: *The Scottish Medical Journal* Online http://www.smj.org.uk/nhs1000.htm).

1990s: The introduction of the 'internal market' applied, it appears, equally to Scotland as to England. [The organisational changes accompanying it, did not. However, organisationally, by 1997 the NHS in Scotland and the NHS in England were very similar, i.e. both had one layer of local statutory authority, acting as 'purchaser' in the internal market—HAs in England, HBs in Scotland. The main difference was that, in England, government control was diffused across 8 regional offices. GP Fundholding was also introduced in Scotland.

1997: The most significant reforms as far as the divergence of the NHS in the UK were those introduced by the Labour government after their election in 1997. The main aim of these reforms, as in England, was the abolition of the competitive structures of the internal market (the purchaser provider split became the strategic/services divide (The NHS in Scotland, Scottish Parliament, 2002). Where they differed from England was largely in the provision of primary care (see Wellards, *NHS Handbook*, 2000/1, 1.2, p. 7). The White Paper, *Designed to Care*, the Scottish counterpart to *The new NHS: modern, dependable*, envisaged two forms of health service trust: Primary Care Trusts (PCTs) and Acute Hospital Trusts (AHTs). PCTs brought together primary, community health and specialist services for the mentally ill, learning disabled and elderly; AHTs merged general hospital services into larger areas of management. This meant that PCTs and AHTs, unlike English PCTs, had no 'commissioning' role (Woods, K., 'Health Policy and the NHS in the UK 1997 – 2002', in *Devolution in Practice*, IPPR, 2002, p. 32), funding for secondary care remaining part of the HB remit. The difference in structural position is illustrated in the fate of GP Fundholding: in Scotland GPs no longer held budgets for the provision of secondary health care, in England the creation of Primary Care Groups (and PCTs), meant that GPs were involved in the commissioning of health services. (In Scotland local healthcare co-operatives were set up to involve GPs in the provisioning of services, but participation in these is voluntary, unlike in England, where all GPs belong to PCTs).

2  Yeun, P. (ed.), *OHE Compendium of Health Statistics*, 14th edn, Office of Health Economics, 2002.

3  Morris (2001) explains that there are 28 NHS Trusts in mainland Scotland covering both acute services and primary care. Trusts were originally constituted as self-governing organisations with boards of executive and non-executive trustees. However, in late 2001 the trust boards were streamlined. They retained their operational and legal  responsibilities within the local health system. 'Trusts have one main financial duty.' 'They obtain most of their income through services agreements with health boards. These agreements set out the treatment or services the trust agrees to provide in return for the funding it is given.' Further income comes from the provision of education and training, including undergraduate and postgraduate doctors and dentists, as well as other income generating schemes such as the sale land. With the exception of Greater Glasgow and Lothian health boards, there is one acute trust (providing A&E, hospital-based surgery and other specialist services) per mainland health board. (Morris, C., 2001, pp. 10-16). The White Paper, *Partnership for Care*, 2003, which announced that all Trusts are to be abolished following legislation which is currently before the Scottish Parliament.

   According to Morris (2001), there are three main elements to the total amount of government expenditure for the NHS in Scotland: SEHD expenditure; centrally managed services expenditure; and hospital and community health services and family health services expenditure. This latter is the largest item including as it does, payments to GPs, dentists, pharmacists and optometrists, as well as the cost of acute and community services. Before funding is allocated to health boards, part of the budget is top-sliced to fund national projects and services such as special health boards and SEHD spending on national programmes (Morris, C., 2001, pp. 15). Health board funding falls into two categories: cash-limited (spent on hospital and community health services (HCHS) including GP prescribing and forming the bulk of the discretionary health board allocation and accounting for some 75% of the total Scottish NHS budget; and non cash-limited (demand-led, spent on family health services provided by doctors (Morris, C., 2001, pp. 15). Since April 2001, HBs have received their income revenue  via the Arbuthnott weighted capitation formula, which reflects the structure and needs of the local population (Morris, C., 2001, pp. 15).

The organisation of primary care in Scotland differs from that in England. 'From April 1999, GPs and staff from mental health, learning disability and other community services, were brought together to form primary care trusts (PCTs). They are responsible for the full range of family health and community services.' PCTs' main tasks are: formulating primary care policy; working in partnership with health boards, acute trusts and others to develop Health Improvement Plans (HIPs); to implement local trust strategies through healthcare co-operatives and to deliver their trust implementation plan; engaging primary and secondary care clinicians in forming agreements and delivering clinical services. They receive their funding from the local health board to cover the cost of GP services. These include GP prescribing and community services, including non-acute hospital services for people with learning disabilities, mental; illness and for frail people.' (Morris, 2001, pp. 12).

Local Health Care Co-operatives (LHCCs) have been established as operational units within PCTs, with responsibility for managing and delivering integrated services across a defined geographical area. They were defined in Designed to Care as: 'voluntary organisations of GPs which will strengthen and support practices in delivering care to their local communities'. In March 2002, there were 82 LHCCs in Scotland (The NHS in Scotland, Scottish Parliament, 2002). GPs not wanting to join an LHCC (of which thee are very few), are allocated a notional budget for prescribing and their share of cash-limited General Medical Services (Community Services are provided for them either by the local co-operative or by the area manager (Scottish Office, *Designed to Care*). The White Paper, *Partnership for Care*, 2003, announced that LHCCs are to be developed in to Community Health Partnerships (CHPs) if legislation before the Scottish Parliament is enacted. For further discussion of primary care in Scotland, see Ritchie, L., 'Developing primary care in Scotland', in Woods, K. and Carter, D., (eds), *Scotland's Health and Health Services*, The Nuffield Trust, 2003.

4   With some minor recent exceptions, patients seldom have the opportunity to exercise effective choice among specialist doctors and hospitals even though (unbeknown to the vast majority, patients do have the right to choose their provider. On 1 July 2002, the English DoH began to make a virtue of the right for patients to travel wherever for treatment when almost 2,000 heart patients who had been waiting six months for an operation became eligible to choose to be treated elsewhere in the NHS or in the private sector. As part of a

pilot, the same choice has been extended to Londoners waiting more than six months for cataract surgery. By early 2003 Londoners waiting for orthopaedic operations, ear, nose and throat treatment, general surgery and other specialities will be able to exercise similar choice. On 3 October 2002, Alan Milburn said that 'if these pilots are successful, choice will be extended to other parts of the country'. Note, in practise, patients have very limited choice of GP. Often, though not always, there is a choice of practice and within an individual practice a choice of GP. However, practicalities often constrain the exercise of choice by patients.

5    Readers should note that the new GP contract (http://www.bma.org.uk/ap.nsf/Content/NewGMScontract/$file/gpcont.pdf ) marks a significant change in the payment system. Until 2003, family doctors in the UK were mainly paid by capitation (payment based on capitation, as opposed to fee-for-service obviates some demand-led prescription) with extra incentive payments for certain services.

   Beyond a minimum practice income, from April 2004, payment will increasingly based on the meeting of quality indicator targets. Published in February 2003, the contract negotiated between the BMA's General Practitioners Committee, the NHS Confederation and the four UK health departments. Aiming to improve the quality of primary care provided by the UK's 42,000 GPs, it has been hailed as the boldest such proposal on this scale ever attempted anywhere in the world (Shekelle, P., 'New contract for general practitioners', *BMJ* 2003;326:457-458 ( 1 March )). 'The proposal spells out 76 quality indicators in 10 clinical domains of care, 56 organisational areas, four assessing patients' experience, and a number of indicators for additional services. The proposal furthermore sets targets for performance that will be accompanied by increased payments to providers.' The contract is likely to increase the cost of prescribing—by up to 10% according to one BMA representative's estimate 92003).Spending on general practice will rise by 33% from £6.1 billion per year to £8 billion by April 2006 (BMA, *New GP contract heralds historic new investment for NHS general practice*, Press Release, BMA London, Friday, 21 Feb 2003).

6    However, choice is a major plank in John Reid's reform plans.

7    Dixon and Robinson, 2002, p. 111.

8    There are also differences between countries in the way waiting times are calculated. (See *Social Trends*, Appendix Part 8 for details).

9  Provider-based hospital waiting lists statistics. These figures
   relate to day case or ordinary admissions—outpatients are not
   included. DoH, Statistical Press notice – NHS Waiting List
   Figures, 30 September 2002, Press release reference: 202/0470,
   Friday 15 November 2002.

10 DoH, Statistical Press notice – NHS Waiting List Figures, 30
   September 2002, Press release reference: 202/0470, Friday 15
   November 2002. 'The total number waiting rose by 12,800
   (1.3%) between September 2001 and September 2002.'

11 ISD, *Annual trends in Activity, Waiting Times and Waiting
   Lists*, figures relate to 'Total on True waiting list'. 'For national
   purposes most inpatient and day case waiting list information
   is recorded at individual patient level on the SMR3 quarterly
   census. The NHSScotland Acute Activity, Waiting Times and
   Waiting Lists site focuses on this list. The national statistics
   sub classify the inpatient and day case waiting lists into three
   categories, i.e. true, deferred admission or planned repeat
   admission waiting lists. The "headline" waiting list figure
   relates to the true waiting list which excludes patients whose
   treatment has been deferred for clinical or personal reasons
   and those waiting for organ transplants (whose limiting factor
   is the availability of organs rather than hospital resources).'
   'The waiting time for inpatient/day case admission is derived
   for all patients who are routinely admitted from the true
   waiting list—admissions via transfer are excluded. The
   waiting time is defined as the difference in days from the date
   the patient was placed on the waiting list to the date of
   admission.' (Source: ISD)

12 (7.22 weeks or 1.67 months) Source: information from
   Directorate of Access & anp; Choice Access Delivery (Waiting
   Times Analysis) Team, 21 March 2003. The median wait, for
   inpatients, day cases and outpatients, is the number of days
   half of the patients will wait less than, and the other half will
   wait more than.

13 Coxon, I. and McCall, A. (eds), *Good Hospital Guide*, *Sunday
   Times*, 6 April 2003, p. 9.

14 ISD, *Annual trends in Activity, waiting Times and Waiting
   Lists*, figures relate to 'Total on True waiting list'. We did not
   find a corresponding figure for England.

15 Coxon, I. and McCall, A. (eds), Good Hospital Guide, the
   *Sunday Times*, 6 April 2003, p. 9.

16  Morris, C., *The Pocket Guide to NHSScotland 2001/2002*, The NHS Confederation, 2001.

17  HPSSS Tables D5 and D6; OHE compendium of statistics; DoH, Hospital.....1991-2001, DoH, 2002; ISD NHSiS resource - online Annual Trends Workforce and Activity. Department of Health HPSSS Table D1; Wellard's NHS Handbook 2001-02, p. 80. Also see: Morris, C., *The Pocket Guide to NHS England*, 2001/2002, The NHS Confederation, 2001.

18  See the NHS Plan and its Scottish equivalent 'Our National Health...'. It is important to differentiate between WTE – whole time equivalents and numbers of staff.

19  Readers should note that many of these tables present data for England *and* Wales. For detailed notes on sources and definitions, see OHE Compendium notes for each table.

## 5: Healthcare Outcomes in England and Scotland

1   In all but the most specialised of fora, Coronary Heart Disease (CHD) and Ischaemic Heart Disease (IHD) are used interchangable. We use CHD in this paper, although a number of our sources use IHD.

2   Thomson, 2002.

3   Source: Leon *et al.*, 2002, Appendix II.

4   Source: Leon *et al.*, 2002, Appendix II and p. 54.

5   Within the group of 17 countries they studied.

6   France and Austria have seen step change improvements for men, while Finland and Spain have seen such improvements for women Leon *et al.*, 2002, pp. 55-57. Considering these findings (and those on cancer survival shown mentioned below), for Denmark, it seems strange that there is so much interest among UK politicians in the Danish health system.

7   Domenighetti and Quaglia, 2001.

8   Phrase from Hurst, 2000.

9   Jee and Or, 1999.

10  OECD, ARD Team, IHD study, 2002. Rates of immunisations, of preventive screening for blood pressure, cholesterol and cancers, the percentage of pregnant women receiving prenatal care in the first trimester, and so forth are other potential indicators (Jee and Or, 1999).

11  See *BMJ* 8 October 2001 for details.

12 See Heart, 'Fifth report on the provision of services for patients with heart disease', Supplement, *Heart*, 2002; 88 (Suppl III): iii1-iii59.

13 Department of Health, *Delivering Better Heart Services – Progress Report: 2003*, NHS 2003.

14 CHD/Stroke task force report, SEHD, 2000. 'International comparisons of Scottish cardiovascular mortality and morbidity rely heavily on data collected in the Glasgow arm of the MONICA study which though of high quality, are not representative of Scotland as a whole'. 'Levels of risk factors for cardiovascular morbidity in Glasgow, with the exception of hypertension, are amongst the highest of all populations in the MONICA study.' Leon *et al.*, p. 28.

15 BHF *Coronary Heart Disease Statistics*, 2003 edition.

16 See BHF *Coronary heart Disease Statistics*, 2003 edition, p. 40.

17 It is not possible to generate incidence rates simply from Hospital Episode Statistics, as these conceal readmissions for CHD. Continuous Morbidity Recording in Scotland employs systems that obviate this difficulty, but these are not used in England.

18 Scottish Executive, The Scottish Health Survey 1998, Scottish Executive Health Department, published November 2000; Department of Health, Health Survey for England 1998, The Stationery Office, December 1999.

19 BHF, statistics 2002, citing Department of Health, *Nutritional Aspects of Cardiovascular Disease*, Report of the Cardio-vascular Disease Review Group of the Committee on Medical Aspects of Food Policy, HMSO: London, 1994.

20 BHF, statistics 2002, citing National Heart Forum, *Coronary heart disease: Estimating the impact of changes in risk factors*, The Stationery Office, 2002.

21 BHF, statistics 2002, pp. 114-127.

22 BHF, statistics 2002. And Leon *et al.*, 2002.

23 These figures must be treated with caution. In order to provide comparable data, only the figures for CABG and PTCA recorded in principal position have been used i.e. only those episodes where the main operation was either PTCA or CABG. Therefore, if somebody was admitted for diagnostic treatment and subsequently received an angioplasty, this would not be counted, for example. This inevitably leads to under reporting,

particularly of PTCAs. This partly explains the disparity between these figures and those provided by the BCIS and SCTS: the BCIS audit gives the total number of PCIs in Scotland in 2000 as 3,007, whereas the ISD give the total as 2,139, a difference of 30 per cent. This is also reflected in the figures for England. The assumption made here is that the difference between operations as main operations and secondary operations is proportionate between England and Scotland. This must be borne in mind when considering this data in comparison with international revascularisation rates, the standards set out in the National Service Framework etc. (Note: the estimates made here are still higher than the NHS Performance indicators for 2002 in England)

24  BCIS audit, 2001 (www. bcis.org.uk/audit/).

25  This is higher than the figures given in the data tables. See note 23 for explanation.

26  This trend was highlighted recently by the OECD ARD team, who posited that some oversupply is owing to economic incentives on providers. Researchers found that the USA, Belgium, Germany and to a lesser extent Australia appear to perform more revascularisations than expected given their relative levels of IHD. The same team found that rates in Italy and Spain appear to reflect IHD levels, but those in Denmark and the UK stand out as being particularly low given levels of IHD (ARD IHD study, p. 13).

27  BCIS audit, 2001 (www.bcis.org.uk/audit/).

28  OPCS4 codes (principal position) – K40 to K46

29  Block, P., Weber, H., Kearney, P., *Manpower in cardiology II in Western and Central Europe* (1997-2000) European Heart Journal, Feb 2003, 22; 4: 299-310.

30  Heart, 'Fifth report on the provision of services for patients with heart disease', Supplement, *Heart*, 2002; 88 (Suppl III): iii1-iii59.

31  BCIS data (www.bcis.org.uk/audit/).

32  Additionally, there are 11 private interventional centres in England and there is one private centre in Glasgow.

33  SCTS National Adult Cardiac Surgical Database Report, 2000-2001.

NOTES 217

34 A number of projects have already been initiated, e.g. the 'Have a Heart Paisley' campaign in Scotland and the National School Fruit Scheme in England.

35 Adab, P. and Rouse, A., 'Is population coronary heart disease risk screening justified? A discussion of the National Service Framework for coronary heart disease (Standard 4)', *British Journal of General Practice*, October 2001: 834-837.

36 'Screening of the whole population for primary prevention purposes would be neither practical nor a cost effective use of health resources. The pick-up rate is likely to be relatively low with a long payback time.'

37 Lipids and the primary prevention of coronary heart disease, SIGN Guidelines 40, September 1999; Shepherd, J., Cobbe, S.M., Ford, I., Isles, C.G., Lorimer, A.R., MacFarlane, P.W. *et al.*, 'Prevention of coronary heart disease with pravastatin in men with hypercholesterolemia. West of Scotland Coronary Prevention Study Group', *N Engl J Med*, 1995; 333: 1301-7; Sacks, F.M., Pfeffer, M.A., Moye, L.A., Rouleau, J.L., Rutherford, J.D., Cole, T.G. *et al.*, 'The effect of pravastatin on coronary events after myocardial infarction in patients with average cholesterol levels. Cholesterol and Recurrent Events Trial investigators', *N Engl J Med*, 1996; 335: 1001-9.

38 Coronary Heart Disease and Stroke task force report, SEHD 2000, p. 41.

39 Wolfe, C. (ed.), McKevitt, C. and Rudd, A., *Stroke Services – Policy and Practice across Europe*, Radcliffe Medical Press, 2002.

40 Bosanquet, N., *Stroke-Reducing the Burden of Disease*, The Stroke Association, 1999.

41 Wolfe, C. *et al.*, for the European Registries of Stroke (EROS) Collaboration, 'Variations in Stroke Incidence and Survival in Three Areas of Europe', *Stroke*, 2000; 31: 2074-2079

42 However, the rate of decline, particularly in younger age-groups, has slowed in recent years. Cf. British Heart Foundation Coronary Heart Disease Statistics, 2003.

43 Sarti, C. *et al.*, 'International Trends in Mortality from Stroke, 1968 to 1994', *Stroke* 2000; 31: 1588-1601.

44 See Wade, D., Mant, J. and Winner, S., 'Stroke - Healthcare Needs Assessment', http://hcna.radcliffe-oxford.com/stroke.htm

45  Death rates for IHD, cancer and cerebrovascular disease were
    compared across the UK countries in the *Registrar General's
    Annual Review of Demographic Trends 2001* but considerable
    doubts were raised by the GRO as to their accuracy after
    publication, largely on account of the lack of age-
    standardisation in the Scottish dataset.

46  Sarti *et al.*, 2000.

47  Leon *et al.*, *Understanding the Health of Scotland's Population
    in an International Context: A review of current approaches,
    knowledge and recommendations for new research directions*,
    Part 1, LSHTM, November 2002, revised, p. 44

48  In Scotland incidence is defined as hospital cases screened
    back to exclude those with previous admissions. In England
    readmissions are not accounted for, making incidence difficult
    to calculate in this way. Moreover, measuring incidence of a
    particular condition according to the Scottish definition is not
    entirely accurate—not all cases result in hospitalisation for
    example.

49  The Oxford Community Stroke Project, the South London
    Stroke Register and the East Lancashire Study in Wade,
    Healthcare Needs Assessment.

50  CMR Monthly Report, *February 1998: Conditions – Stroke*, ISD
    Scotland, May 1998.

51  Syme, P., Byrne, A., Devenny, R., Chen, R. and Forbes, J., 'The
    community-based incidence of Stroke in a Scottish population',
    the Scottish Borders Stroke Study (SBSS), presented at the
    European Stroke Conference, Valencia, May 2003,
    *CHD / Stroke Task Force Report*, SEHD, 2000.

52  Health Survey for England 1998; Scottish Health Survey 1998.

53  Wolfe, C. *et al.*, 2001.

54  Source: OECD, ARD Team, 2002.

55  OECD, ARD Team, Stroke study, 2002, p. 6.

56  Wolfe, C. *et al.*, for the European BIOMED Study of Stroke
    Care Group, 'Variations in Case Fatality and Dependency
    From Stroke in Western and Central Europe', *Stroke*, 1999;
    30: 350-356.

57  Wolfe, C. *et al.*, 2000.

58 Weir, N. *et al.*, on behalf of the IST Collaborative Group, 'Variations Between Countries in Outcome after Stroke in the International Stroke Trial', *Stroke*, 2001; 32: 1370-1377.

59 Source: OECD, ARD Team, 2002.

60 OECD, ARD Team, Stroke study, 2002, p. 19.

61 OECD, ARD Team, Stroke study, 2002, p. 11, figure 5.

62 Langthorne, P. *et al.*, Collaborative systematic review of the randomised trials of organised inpatient (stroke unit) care after stroke, *BMJ* 1997; 314: 1151.

63 The Stroke Association, *Stroke Care – A Matter of Chance*, A National Survey of Stroke Services, 1999.

64 Langthorne, P. (ed.) and Dennis, M., *Stroke Units: An Evidence Based Approach*, BMJ Books, 1998.

65 Lindley *et al.*, 'Hospital services for patients with acute stroke in the United Kingdom: the Stroke Association survey of consultant opinion', *Age Ageing*, 1995; 24: 525-532.

66 Grieve, R. *et al.*, on behalf of the European BIOMED II European Study of Stroke Care, 'A Comparison of the Costs and Survival of Hospital-admitted Stroke Patients across Europe', *Stroke* 2001; 32: 1684-1691.

67 OECD, ARD Team, Stroke Study, 2002, p. 9.

68 *Summary Report on the National Sentinel Stroke Audit 2001-02*, Royal College of Physicians of London, July 2002.

69 Dennis, M., (University of Edinburgh), personal communication, 2003.

70 Roberts, M. *et al.*, 'Organisation of services for acute stroke in Scotland – report of the Scottish stroke services audit', *Health Bulletin* 58 (2) March 2000.

71 Royal College of Physicians, *The National Sentinel Audit of Stroke 1998-99*.

72 OECD, ARD Team, Stroke study 2002.

73 Royal College of Physicians, *National Sentinel Stroke Audit 2001-02*.

74 Scottish Executive, *Coronary Heart Disease and Stroke – Strategy for Scotland*, Appendix, SEHD 2001.

75  According to Health Statistics Quarterly 17, HSQ 18 was due to include an article entitled: 'Atlas of cancer indicators and mortality in the United Kingdom and Ireland'. Unfortunately no such article appeared.

76  Johnston, P. and McDermott, U., *The Principles and Practice of Oncology*, Citing Berrino *et al.*, 1995.

77  Johnston and McDermott, *The Principles and Practice of Oncology*, citing Berrino *et al.*, 1995.

78  Johnston and McDermott, *The Principles and Practice of Oncology*, citing Berrino *et al.*, 1995.

79  Calman-Hine Report (Department of Health, Chief Medical Officer's Expert Advisory Group on Cancer, *A Policy Framework for Commissioning Cancer Services*, London: Department of Health, 1995).

80  Sikora, K., 'Rationing cancer care', in *The Realities of Rationing*, 1999.

81  Sikora, 'Rationing cancer care', 1999, pp. 134-35.

82  Green, D.G. and Caspar, L., *Delay, Denial, Dilution*, Choice in Welfare No 55, IEA Health and Welfare Unit, 2000, citing Sikora, 'Rationing cancer care', 1999.

83  Department of Health, *Health of the Nation* cited in Coleman, M., Babb, P. *et al.*, *Cancer survival trends in England and Wales, 1971-1995: deprivation and NHS Region*, ONS, Studies in Medical and Population Subjects, No. 61, London: TSO, 1999.

84  Department of Health, *Saving Lives: Our Healthier Nation*, Cm.4386, London: TSO, July 1999, p. 61.

85  Department of Health, *The NHS Cancer Plan, 2000*, pp. 48-54. Also see *The NHS Cancer Plan – Making Progress*. On 7 March 2003 Health minister Hazel Blears addressed a cancer conference in Birmingham. She said that the government wants to reduce the period from diagnosis to treatment to just four weeks.

86  This pledge followed research findings reported in the *BMJ* in April 1999. After reviewing 87 worldwide studies 'researchers at Guy's and St Thomas's Hospital, London, found that five year survival rates were 12 per cent lower among women whose treatment did not begin until three months or more after their first symptom appeared.

87 Mayor S., 'Review of cancer services shows poor coordination in NHS', *BMJ* 2001;323:1383

88 Department of Health, *Building on Experience, Breast Screening Programme Annual Review 2002*, NHS, 2002.

89 Part of a letter from the national Cancer Director (dubbed Cancer Tsar), Professor Mike Richards, to all Health Authorities and PCTs, cancer network managers. The funding is intended to enable one session per week to be released for the role of Primary Care Cancer Lead.

90 The NHS Modernisation Board, *The Annual Report (2003) of the NHS Modernisation Board*.

91 Mayor, S., 'UK improves cancer control', *BMJ* 2003;326:72.

92 The NHS Modernisation Board, *The Annual Report (2003) of the NHS Modernisation Board*, 2003, p. 2.

93 Royal College of Radiologists, *Medical Manpower and Workload in Clinical Oncology*, 1991.

94 Green, D.G. and Caspar, L., *Delay, Denial, Dilution*, Choice in Welfare No 55, IEA Health and Welfare Unit, 2000, citing Sikora, 'Rationing cancer care', in *The Realities of Rationing*, 1999, pp. 134-35.

95 NHS Modernisation Board, *The Annual Report (2003) of the NHS Modernisation Board*, March 2003.

96 Forrest, P.A.M., *Breast Cancer Screening, report to Health Ministers of England, Wales, Scotland and Northern Ireland by a working group*, HMSO, 1987.

97 A mammography is an x-ray of each breast.

98 Scottish Executive Health Department, *Cancer Scenarios*, SCG, 2001; DoH, *Building on Experience, Breast Screening Programme Annual Review 2002*, NHS, 2002.

99 The NHS Modernisation Board, *The Annual Report (2003) of the NHS Modernisation Board*, 2003.

100 One from above and one from the armpit. Research shows that this could improve detection rates of small cancers by up to 43 per cent (The Cancer Plan).

101 Mayor, S., 'Review of cancer services shows poor coordination in NHS', *BMJ* 2001;323:1383.

102 Sikora, K., Speech to Reform Britain conference, 7 April 2003.

103  Johnston, P. and McDermott, U., *The Principles and Practice of Oncology*, citing Berrino *et al.*, 1995. Also see Coleman, M., Babb, P. *et al.*, *Cancer survival trends in England and Wales, 1971-1995: deprivation and NHS Region*, ONS, Studies in Medical and Population Subjects, No. 61, London: The Stationery Office, 1999.

104  Audit Commission and CHI, *NHS Cancer Care in England and Wales*, London: The Stationery Office, 2001.

105  Audit Commission and CHI, *NHS Cancer Care in England and Wales*, London: The Stationery Office, 2001.

106  Figures published on Friday 7 March 2003. Reported by BBC online.

107  Audit Commission and CHI, *NHS Cancer Care in England and Wales*, The Stationery Office, 2001.

108  Audit Commission and CHI, *NHS Cancer Care in England and Wales*, The Stationery Office, 2001; Mayor, S., 'Review of cancer services shows poor coordination in NHS', *BMJ* 2001;323:1383.

109  Coleman, M., Babb, P. *et al.*, *Cancer survival trends in England and Wales, 1971-1995: deprivation and NHS Region*, ONS, Studies in Medical and Population Subjects, No. 61, London: The Stationery Office, 1999.

110  NCEPOD, 2001.

111  Source: Scottish Executive, *Cancer in Scotland: Action for Change*. Page 2 of the summary of the New White Paper, *Partnerships for Care*, again highlights the fact that Scotland has 'some of the highest death rates in the world for cancer and heart disease'.

112  Scottish Health on the Web: www.show.nhs.uk/isd/cancer/cancer.htm

113  Scottish Executive, *Cancer in Scotland: Action for Change* [Glossary], 2001.

114  Scottish Executive, *Cancer in Scotland: Action for Change* [Glossary], 2001.

115  Scottish Executive Health Department, *Cancer Scenarios: An aid to planning cancer services in Scotland in the next decade*, The Scottish Executive, Edinburgh, 2001.

116  Sometimes referred to as Scottish Cancer Strategy.

117  Scottish Executive, *Cancer in Scotland: Action for Change*.

118 Scottish Executive, *Cancer in Scotland: Action for Change*, p. 24.

119 Scottish Executive, *Cancer in Scotland: Action for Change*, p. 24.

120 Scottish Executive, *Cancer in Scotland: Action for Change*, p. 25.

121 Scottish Executive, *Our National Health: a plan for action, a plan for change*, see pp. 37-48.

122 Scottish Executive, NHSScotland, *Scottish Referral Guidelines for Suspected Cancer*, Scottish Executive, 2002. 'An individual GP is likely to see no more that 7 or 8 new cases per annum.' The average number of new cases p.a. of lung cancer for a GP with a list size of 1,500 patients (the average list size in Scotland) is about one or two. 'An individual GP will also see about one new patient with breast cancer and on with colorectal cancer per annum, but will only see about one new case of ovarian cancer once every five years and a new case of testicular cancer every 20 years' (p. 3).

123 The five cancer centres were predetermined solely by the presence of linear accelerators; unlike England, Scotland has not designated 'cancer centres' or 'cancer units'.

124 Scottish Executive, *Cancer in Scotland: Action for Change*, p. 29.

125 MCN's might be disease or specialty-based.

126 SCAN, *Annual Report 2001-2*, South East Scotland Cancer Network, 2002.

127 Scottish Executive, *Cancer in Scotland: Action for Change*, p. 29.

128 Minutes of reformed SCG, July 2001.

129 Since 1997, cancer registration has used the SOCRATES system.

130 Scottish Executive, *Cancer in Scotland: Action for Change*, p. 11. Also note the 1996 Diet Action Plan for Scotland, *Eating for Health*, and the 1999 White Paper, *Towards a Healthier Scotland*.

131 Scottish Executive, *Cancer in Scotland: Action for Change*, p. 11.

132  Scottish Executive, *Cancer in Scotland: Action for Change*, p. 12.

133  Scottish Executive, *Plan for Action on Alcohol Problems*, January 2002. In 1998, 33 per cent of men exceeded the 21 units per week recommended consumption—a rate unchanged from 1995. The rates for women (whose recommended maximum in 14 units per week) are lower, but are increasing; from 13 per cent in 1995 to 15 per cent in 1998. Alcohol misuse costs the NHS in Scotland something approaching £90 million (derived from Guest, J. and Varney, S., *Alcohol Misuse in Scotland: Trends and Costs*, Catalyst Health Economic Consultants Ltd).

134  Scottish Executive, *Cancer in Scotland: Action for Change*, p. 29.

135  Scottish Executive, *Cancer in Scotland: Action for Change*, p. 25.

136  Scottish Executive, *Our National Health: A plan for action, a plan for change*, p. 41.

137  2002/03: £15 million. 2003/04: £15 million. Source: minutes of reformed SCG, July 2001.

138  Scottish Breast Screening Programme. ISD Online.

139  Scottish Executive, *Cancer in Scotland: Action for Change*, p. 20.

140  Scottish Breast Screening Programme. ISD Online.

141  In light of UK Screening Committee recommendations, in 2000 the SE established a Demonstration Project—The Cancer Challenge—to see if screening for colorectal cancer is feasible and publicly acceptable (Scottish Executive, *Cancer in Scotland: Action for Change*, p. 20).

142  The level of prostate specific antigen (PSA) in the blood may be investigated to confirm diagnosis, but this is not currently recommended by the UK Screening Committee (*Cancer in Scotland: Action for Change*, p. 20).

143  Report from 12 December 2002. http://news.bbc.co.uk/1/hi/Scotland/2569943.stm (accessed on 7 March 2003).

144  CRC, About Cancer Statistics (webdoc).

145  The EUROCARE II study presents comparable, population-based cancer survival statistics of 3.5 million cancer patients from 1985-1989. Data from 17 countries were collected, including: Iceland, Finland, Sweden, Denmark, Scotland, England, The Netherlands, Germany, Austria, Switzerland, France, Spain, Italy, Slovenia, Slovakia, Poland, and Estonia.

146  See: Cookson, J.B., 'Cancer survival', [Letter] *Lancet* 356(9241):1611, 4 November 2000; Woodman, C.B., Gibbs, A., Scott, N., Haboubi, N.Y. and Collins, S., 'Are differences in stage at presentation a credible explanation for reported differences in the survival of patients with colorectal cancer in Europe?', *British Journal of Cancer*, 85(6):787-90, 14 September 2001; Prior, P., Woodman, C.B. and Collins, S., 'International differences in survival from colon cancer: more effective care versus less complete cancer registration', *British Journal of Surgery*, 85(1):101-4, January 1998.

147  Prior, *et al.*, 1998.

148  Woodman *et al.*, 'Are differences in stage at presentation a credible explanation for reported differences in the survival of patients with colorectal cancer in Europe?', *British Journal of Cancer*, 2001; Cookson, 'Cancer survival', [Letter] *Lancet*, 2000; Prior, Woodman and Collins, 'International differences in survival from colon cancer: more effective care versus less complete cancer registration' *British Journal of Surgery*, 1998; Gatta, G., Capocaccia, R. and Berrino, F., 'Cancer survival differences between European populations: the UK uneasiness', [comment], [Comment. Editorial] *British Journal of Cancer*, 85(6):785-6, 14 September 2001.

149  Gatta, Capocaccia and Berrino, 'Cancer survival differences between European populations: the UK uneasiness' *British Journal of Cancer*, 2001.

150  Cookson, 'Cancer survival', *Lancet*, 2000.

151  Forman, D., Gatta, G., Capocaccia, R., Janssen-Heijnen, M.L. and Coebergh, J.W., 'Cancer survival', [Comment, Letter] *Lancet*, 357(9255):555, 17 February 2001.

152  EUROCARE II; and Coleman, M. *et al.*, *Cancer Survival Trends in England and Wales, 1971-1995: deprivation and NHS Region*, The Stationery Office, 1999, p. 102.

153  ISD Scotland, *Trends in Cancer Survival Scotland: 1971-1995*.

154  CRC, About Cancer Statistics (webdoc).

155  Coleman, M., Babb, P. *et al.*, *Cancer Survival Trends in England and Wales, 1971-1995: deprivation and NHS Region*, ONS, Studies in Medical and Population Subjects, No. 61, London: The Stationery Office, 1999.

156  This overall trend does not apply in each and every cancer site.

157  The term 'All cancers' refers to cancers overall, rather than each and every cancer.

158  From Quinn, Babb *et al.*, *Cancer Trends in England and Wales 1950-1999*, 2001.

159  Quinn, Babb *et al.*, *Cancer Trends in England and Wales 1950-1999*, 2001.

160  http://www.show.scot.nhs.uk/isd/cancer/facts_figures/facts_figures.htm  Accessed on 10 April 2003.

161  Quinn, Babb *et al.*, *Cancer Trends in England and Wales 1950-1999*, 2001.

162   Coleman, Babb *et al.*, *Cancer Survival Trends in England and Wales, 1971-1995: deprivation and NHS Region*, 1999 (England and Wales age standardisation population—see pages 48-50 of source).

163  CRC, About Cancer Statistics (webdoc).

164  Quinn, Babb *et al.*,*Cancer Trends 1950-99*, p. 84.

165  The NHS Modernisation Board, *The Annual Report (2003) of the NHS Modernisation Board*, 2003.

166  CRAG, *Clinical Outcomes Indicators*, Clinical Resource and Audit Group, Scottish Executive, 2002. Leon *et al.*, (pp. 50-51) examined lung cancer mortality by age and year of birth. Their findings revealed very similar patterns between England and Scotland. Male's peak lung cancer mortality was earlier (those born 1901-05) than that for women (those born 1920-24). Though patterns are similar, rates increased further in Scotland. Leon posits that this is perhaps because of the later emergence of smoking cessation and the low consumption of fruit and vegetables.

167  CRAG, *Clinical Outcomes Indicators*, Clinical Resource and Audit Group, Scottish Executive, 2002.

168 Danish women, who also smoke unusually heavily, have similarly high incidence and mortality rates. Leon *et al.*, 2002, p. 42.

169 CRAG, *Clinical Outcomes Indicators*, Clinical Resource and Audit Group, Scottish Executive, 2002, pp. 68-77.

170 CRC, About Cancer Statistics (webdoc).

171 Leon *et al.*, 2002, p. 42.

172 Quinn, Babb *et al.*, *Cancer Trends 1950-99*, p. 41.

173 Quinn, Babb *et al.*, *Cancer Trends 1950-99*, p. 40.

174 Quinn, *et al.*, 1998.

175 OECD ARD team, 'Summary of Results from Breast Cancer Disease Study', 2002.

176 Green, D. and Irvine, B. (eds), *They've Had a Good Innings*, Civitas, 2003.

177 Brown, P., 'UK death rates from breast cancer fall by a third', *BMJ*, 2000;321:849.

178 Sir Richard Peto, quoted by Brown, P., 'UK death rates from breast cancer fall by a third', *BMJ*, 2000;321:849. Also see *Trends in Cancer Survival Scotland: 1975-95*, Chapter 12.

179 Brown, P., 'UK death rates from breast cancer fall by a third', *BMJ*, 2000.

180 ISD Scotland, *Trends in Cancer Survival in Scotland: 1971-95*, Chapter 12.

181 Gatta, Faivre, *et al.*, 1998.

182 Janice Hopkins reports that cancer mortality in the US may be underrecorded because deaths within a month of surgery for solid tumours are recorded as deaths related to treatment. Researchers estimated the proportion of deaths not attributed to cancer for 19 common solid tumours. Cancer was not recorded as the cause of death for 42 per cent of 1,695 colorectal cancer patients, 34 per cent of 525 lung cancer patients, 54 per cent of 265 bladder cancer patients, 24 per cent of ovarian cancer patients, and 75 per cent of prostate cancer patients (Hopkins, J., *BMJ* 2002; 325: 182).

183 ISD Scotland, *Trends in Cancer Survival in Scotland: 1971-95*, Chapters 5 and 6; and Quinn and Babb *et al.*, *Cancer Trends 1950-99*, p. 55.

184 ISD Scotland, *Trends in Cancer Survival in Scotland: 1971-95*, Chapters 5 and 6; and Quinn and Babb *et al.*, *Cancer Trends 1950-99*.

185 CRC, About Cancer Statistics (webdoc). ISD Scotland, *Trends in Cancer Survival in Scotland: 1971-95*, Chapter 16; and Quinn and Babb *et al.*, *Cancer Trends 1950-99*.

186 Quinn and Babb *et al.*, *Cancer Trends 1950-99*, p. 127.

187 Post *et al.*, 1998.

188 ISD Scotland, *Trends in Cancer Survival in Scotland: 1971-95*, Chapter 16; Quinn and Babb *et al.*, *Cancer Trends 1950-99*, p. 127.

189 Quinn and Babb *et al.*, *Cancer Trends 1950-99*, p. 46.

190 ISD Scotland, *Trends in Cancer Survival in Scotland: 1971-95*, Chapter 13; Quinn and Babb *et al.*, *Cancer Trends 1950-99*, p. 148.

191 Gatta, Lasota, *et al.*, 1998.

192 Gatta, Lasota, *et al.*, 1998, note that in countries characterised by relatively poor survival for cervical cancer at the end of the 1970s, five-year survival increased at a greater rate than the European average; this was particularly evident in England and Scotland.

193 ISD Scotland, *Trends in Cancer Survival in Scotland: 1971-95*, Chapter 13.

194 Quinn and Babb *et al.*, *Cancer Trends 1950-99*, p. 138.

195 Johnston, P., McDermott, U., *The Principles and Practice of Oncology*, citing Berrino *et al.*, 1995.

196 CHI/Audit commission, NSF Assessments, Supporting Data, No. 1, 2001, pp. 11-17.

197 Source: Berrino, F., EUROCARE II Study, 1999.

198 Sikora, *Cancer Survival in Britain*, 1999.

199 The NHS Modernisation Board, *The Annual Report (2003) of the NHS Modernisation Board*, 2003, pp. 1-15.

200 The NHS Modernisation Board, *The Annual Report (2003) of the NHS Modernisation Board*, 2003, pp. 1-15.

201 The NHS Modernisation Board, *The Annual Report (2003) of the NHS Modernisation Board*, 2003, pp. 1-15.

202 Scottish Executive, *Cancer in Scotland: Action for Change*, p. 24.

203 Scottish Executive, *Cancer in Scotland: Action for Change*, p. 24; Scottish Executive, Scottish Cancer Group, *Cancer in Scotland: Action for Change, Annual Report 2002*, 2002.

204 Scottish Executive, *Cancer in Scotland: Action for Change, Annual Report 2002*, 2002.

205 Department of Health, *A Survey of Radiotherapy Services in England, 1999*. Also see 2001 report.

206 The NHS Modernisation Board, *The Annual Report (2003) of the NHS Modernisation Board*, 2003, p. 4.

207 NHS Modernisation Board, *The Annual Report (2003) of the NHS Modernisation Board*, 2003.

208 2002/03: £15 million. 2003/04: £15 million. Source: minutes of reformed SCG, July 2001.

209 Scottish Executive, *Cancer in Scotland: Action for Change, Annual Report 2002*, 2002.

210 Scottish Executive, *Cancer in Scotland: Action for Change, Annual Report 2002*, 2002.

211 Christie, B., 'Cancer Centre at "breaking point"', *BMJ* 2001;328:1148.

212 Christie, 'Cancer Centre at "breaking point"', *BMJ*, 2001.

213 Christie, 'Cancer Centre at "breaking point"', *BMJ*, 2001.

214 Gregor, A., 'Foreword', *Cancer in Scotland: Action for Change, National Implementation Plan 2002/03*, 2002.

215 Scottish Executive Health Department, NHSScotland, *Cancer Scenarios*, 2001, Chapter 24. Other procedures are used for certain cancers (e.g. Selectron units and HDR machines and Brachytherapy).

216 Department of Health, *A Survey of Radiotherapy Services in England*, 1999, p. 42.
p. 42.

217 'The administration of radiotherapy changed significantly during the 1950s with the development of megavoltage radiotherapy treatment machines. ... Two kinds of machines were developed which are still in widespread use. Linear accelerators which generate high energy x-rays and electrons using electricity, and Cobalt unit which use a radioactive

source of high-energy gamma rays. Linear accelerators are more expensive (approximately £1 M) and require specialist support to keep them running in a safe and effective manner. Cobalt units are less expensive, more reliable and easier to maintain than linear accelerators. However, cobalt units produce a radiation beam of a lower energy than modern linear accelerators and also have inferior beam geometry. In addition, cobalt units are associated with the risks of accidental radiation exposure, which could result from a mechanical failure or fire, and the problems associated with the disposal of a spent radioactive source.' DoH, *A Survey of Radiotherapy Services in England*, 1999, p. 42.

218  Hughes, M., OECD, 2003.

219  Hughes, M., OECD, 2003, p. 89.

220  Hughes, M., OECD, 2003, p. 89.

221  Hughes, M., OECD, 2003.

222  Hughes, M., OECD, 2003, p. 89.

223  Scottish Executive Health Department, NHSScotland, *Cancer Scenarios*, 2001, p. 308.

224  Department of Health, *The NHS Plan Implementation Programme*, 2000, p. 15.

225  The NHS Modernisation Board, *The Annual Report (2003) of the NHS Modernisation Board*, 2003.

226  This figure is due to rise to 24 in the next couple of years (Source: Scottish executive personal communication, March 2003).

227  CHI / Audit commission (3.19-3.21), 2001.

228  CHI / Audit commission (3.22), 2001.

229  NHSScotland, *Cancer Scenarios*, Chapters 24-25.

230  Royal College of Radiologists, *Equipment, Workload and Staffing for Radiotherapy in Scotland*, London: Royal college of Radiologists, 2000.

231  Royal College of Radiologists, *Equipment, Workload and Staffing for Radiotherapy in Scotland*, 2000.

232  Department of Health, *Vacancies Survey*, DoH 2002.

233  Royal College of Radiologists, *Clinical Radiology: A Workforce in Crisis*, London: Royal College of Radiologists, 2002.

234  Lack of treatment protocols may also serve to explain variations across countries in survival.

235  OECD, ARD Team, 'Summary of Breast Cancer Disease Study, 2002.

236  Mayor, S., 'Study confirms that screening reduces deaths from breast cancer', *BMJ* 2001;322:1140. The study referred to showed that mortality from incident breast carcinoma diagnosed in women aged 40-69 years fell by 63 per cent in those who were screened during the period when mammography was available (1988-96) compared with the period when it was not (1968-77).

237  The IARC convened an international panel of 24 experts in Lyon in March 2002, to review trial evidence of the efficacy of mammography (Source: DoH, *Building on Experience, Breast Screening Programme Annual Review 2002*, NHS, 2002).

238  DoH, *Building on Experience, Breast Screening Programme Annual Review 2002*, NHS, 2002.

239  DoH, *Breast Screening Programme England: Bulletin 2001-02*, February 2003.

240  DoH, *Breast Screening Programme England: Bulletin 2000-01*, 2002, pp. 1-5.

241  DoH, *Breast Screening Programme England: Bulletin 2000-01*, 2002, pp. 1-5.

242  DoH, *Breast Screening Programme England: Bulletin 2001-02*, February 2003.

243  DoH, *Breast Screening Programme England: Bulletin 2000-01*, 2002, pp. 1-5.

244  DoH, *Breast Screening Programme England: Bulletin 2001-02*, February 2003.

245  OECD, ARD Team, 'Summary of Results from Breast Cancer Disease Study, 2002.

246  Scottish Breast Screening Programme. ISD Online.

247  DoH, *Building on Experience, Breast Screening Programme Annual Review 2002*, NHS, 2002, p. 21.

248  OECD, ARD Team, 'Summary of results from Breast Cancer Disease Study', 2002.

249  DoH, *NHS Cancer Plan*, p. 34.

250 DoH, *Cervical Screening Programme England: Bulletin 2002/21*, October 2002. 'The information for this publication is collected on three Department of Health returns. Information form the call and recall system is collected on return KC53. Information about cervical smears examined by pathology laboratories is collected on return KC61 ... Information of referrals to coloscopy, whether following a smear or clinical indication, and subsequent treatment is collected on return KC65; 2001-02 was the first year of mandatory collection of this return.'

251 A pilot of a new cervical screening technique using liquid based cytology has already taken place. (Scottish Executive, *Cancer in Scotland: Action for Change*, p. 19.) Similar pilots have taken place in England following a recommendation of NICE.

252 Scottish Executive, *Cancer in Scotland: Action for Change*, p. 19.

253 Scottish Executive, *Cancer in Scotland: Action for Change*, p. 19.

254 Cervical Cytology Statistics are collected quarterly from laboratories (on form ISD(D)1Q) and annually from health boards (on form ISD(D)4). The data are compiled by the Hospital and Community Information Unit (HCIU) in ISD Scotland.

255 England: DoH, *Cervical Screening Programme England: Bulletin 2002/21*, October 2002, Table 2.

256 England: DoH, *Cervical Screening Programme England: Bulletin 2002/21*, October 2002, Table 2.

257 Johnston, P., McDermott, U., *The Principles and Practice of Oncology*, citing Berrino *et al.*, 1995.

258 OECD, ARD Team, 'Summary of Results from Breast Cancer Disease Study', 2002. Also see Hughes, M., 2003 in OECD, ARD Team, 2003.

259 OECD, ARD Team, 'Summary of Results from Breast Cancer Disease Study', 2002, pp. 4-7. Also see Hughes, M., 2003 in OECD, ARD Team, 2003.

260 OECD, ARD Team, 'Summary of Results from Breast Cancer Disease Study', 2002, p. 18. Also see Hughes, M., 2003 in OECD, ARD Team, 2003.

261 OECD, ARD Team, 'Summary of Results from Breast Cancer Disease Study', 2002, pp. 18-19. The average of 28 per cent excludes figures for individual Canadian Provinces. Also see Hughes, M., 2003 in OECD, ARD Team, 2003.

262 OECD, ARD Team, 'Summary of Results from Breast Cancer Disease Study', 2002, p. 20. Also see Hughes, M., 2003 in OECD, ARD Team, 2003.

263 Hughes, 2003 in OECD, ARD Team, 2003.

264 Hughes, 2003 in OECD, ARD Team, 2003.

265 OECD, ARD Team, 'Summary of Results from Breast Cancer Disease Study, 2002.

266 OECD, ARD Team, 'Summary of Results from Breast Cancer Disease Study, 2002.

267 OECD, ARD Team, 'Summary of Results from Breast Cancer Disease Study, 2002, citing Mandelblatt, *et al.*, 'Measuring and predicting surgeons' practice styles for breast cancer treatment in older women', *Medical Care*, Vol. 39 (3), 2001, pp. 228-242.

268 Hughes, 2003 in OECD, ARD Team, 2003.

269 Gregor, A. *et al.*, 'Management and survival of patients with lung cancer in Scotland diagnosed in 1995: results of a national population based study', *Thorax* 2001; 56: 212-217.

270 *BMJ* Editorial, 'Thoracic surgery in a crisis', *BMJ* 2002; 324:376-77. Also see 'The Critical Underprovision of Thoracic Surgery in the UK', Report of a joint Working Group of the British Thoracic Society and the Society of Cardiothoracic Surgeons of Great Britain and Ireland, (Draft, 2001).

271 Janssen-Heijnen *et al.*, 1998.

272 'The Critical Underprovision of Thoracic Surgery in the UK', Report of a joint Working Group of the British Thoracic Society and the Society of Cardiothoracic Surgeons of Great Britain and Ireland, (Draft, 2001).

273 The percentage of cases which have been verified histologically is a positive indicator of the validity of diagnosis. The higher the proportion of histological verification, the more confident one can be that a neoplasm existed and that it was primary rather than metastatic. Also, NYCRIS, Cancer Outcomes monitoring, Leeds, 1999.

274 Janssen-Heijnen *et al.*, 1998.

275  Melling *et al.*, 'Lung cancer referral patterns in the former Yorkshire region of the UK', *British Journal of Cancer*, 2002; 86: 36-42.

276  Janssen-Heijnen *et al.*, 1998, citing, Gatta, G. and Sant, M., (on behalf of the EUROCARE working group) 'Patterns of treatment of lung cancer patients in Europe (abstract)', 1993 annual meeting of the International Association of Cancer Registries, Bratislava, Slovakia, 1993.

277  NYCRIS, Cancer Outcomes monitoring, Leeds, 1999. Also Gregor *et al*, 2001.

## 6: Discussion

1  Dixon, J., *What is the hard evidence on the performance of "mainstream" health services serving deprived compared to non-deprived areas in England?*, Report for the Social Exclusion Unit, September 2000.

2  The link between expenditure and outcomes is much more significant for women than for men. (Or, 2000A) considers that this difference in impact on health outcomes may be owing to differences in mortality patterns. Male mortality rates seem less sensitive to medical intervention. 'In most OECD countries, around 30 per cent of the premature mortality for men is a result of "external causes" such as violence, accidents', while for women, cancer is the leading cause of death, accounting for between 20 and 30 per cent, with 'external cause' represent only about 16 per cent. Women also benefit from a number of systematic prevention programmes such as screening for cancer (Or, 2000A).

3  Or, 2000A and Domenighetti and Quaglia 2001. Domenighetti and Quaglia note that infant mortality is correlated with health expenditure. Certain other simple correlations between expenditure and other indicators can be observed: The higher expenditure, the higher the number of beds per 1,000, and the greater the length of stays. These two factors do not necessarily affect medical outcomes.

   Perhaps observing the diminishing returns, and outlying performers (such as Sweden and the US, the latter was not included in their study), Domenighetti and Quaglia find that avoidable mortality, owing to medical intervention (with or without the inclusion of CHD), is not correlated with health expenditure.

4  See Or, 2000; and OECD various.

5 In their study of 2001, Domenighetti and Quaglia found the best performing country to be Sweden, which with expenditure of $1,701 per capita, and reveals the best group of indicators— at the top of the scale. The worst performing country from health perspective was found to be the UK—which has a group of indicators at the bottom of the scale.

6 Although the existence of iatrogenic disease (med.(of illness or symptoms) induced in a patient as the result of a physician's words or action (Collins definition)—the concept is directly related to supplier-induced healthcare demand) should be recalled—particularly for systems where fee-for service payment is used.

7 Domenighetti and Quaglia, 2001.

8 Grubaugh and Santerre, 1994.

9 Domenighetti and Quaglia, 2001; and Or, 2000.

10 Feachem, R.G.A., Sekhri, N.K. and White., K.L., 'Getting more for their dollar: a comparison of the NHS with California's Kaiser Permanente', *BMJ* 2002;324:135-143 ( 19 January ).

11 It is worth noting that despite concerns, the government, guided by the Strategy Unit of the DoH, has taken on board lessons from Kaiser Permanente on chronic disease management. For detail see: http://www.natpact.nhs.uk/chronic_disease_management/kaiser.php

12 Leon *et al.*, p. 28.

13 See Hanlon, P. *et al.*, *Chasing the Scottish Effect: why Scotland needs a step-change in health if it is to catch up with the rest of Europe*, Public Health Institute of Scotland, 2001.

14 Leon, D., Morton, S., Cannegieter, S., McKee, M., *Understanding the Health of Scotland's Population in an International Context: A review of current approaches, knowledge and recommendations for new research directions*, Part 1, LSHTM, November 2002, (revised).

15 Carstairs, V., Morris, R., 'Deprivation: explaining differences in mortality between Scotland, England and Wales', *BMJ* 1989; 299:886-9. Also see: Carstairs, V., Morris, R., *Deprivation and Health in Scotland*, Aberdeen: Aberdeen University Press, 1991.

16 'Using the Carstairs and Morris method of categorising deprivation', Hanlon, P. *et al.*, (2001), show that 'in 1991, 18 per cent of the Scottish population were deemed to be living in

areas of high deprivation (categories 6 and 7) compared to nine per cent in England and Wales'. Some '52 per cent of the "worst of million" people in the UK in terms of health live in Scotland'. (Blamey *et al.*, 2002, citing Shaw, M., Dorling, D., Gordon, D. and Davey Smith, G., *The Widening Gap: Health Inequalities and policy in Britain*,1999.)

17  Griffiths, C. and Fitzpatrick, J., *Geographic Variations in Health*, DS No. 16, London: HMSO, 2001.

18  Leon, Morton, Cannegieter and McKee, *Understanding the Health of Scotland's Population in an International Context*, 2002, pp. 65-66.

19  Leon, *et al.*, 2002, p. 66.

20  Leon, *et al.*, 2002, p. 67.

21  See Blamey, A., Hanlonm P., Judge, K. and Murie, J. (eds), *Health Inequalities in the New Scotland*, PHIS, 2002, p. 19. In the early 1990s, deprivation accounted for roughly 40 per cent of excess deaths at all ages. Also see See Hanlon, P. *et al.*, *Chasing the Scottish Effect: why Scotland needs a step-change in health if it is to catch up with the rest of Europe*, PHIS, 2001.

22  Leon, *et al.*, 2002. p. 5.

23  Leon, *et al.*, 2002. pp. 5-13.

24  Leon *et al.*, 2002, pp. 5-13. Outcomes in Wales and Northern Ireland, generally tend to be worse that those in England.

25  OECD, *Health Data*, 2002. Also OECD, *Health Data*, 2003.

26  Making a connection between a funding system, expenditure, and medical outcomes is fraught with difficulty. The chief problem is that no country has a single system of finance, whereas outcome data are presented for the whole country. We cannot, therefore, be entirely sure whether favourable outcomes are due to the public or private elements of any arrangements. Moreover, competition may be driving performance rather than the funding mechanism and two national systems based on the same funding model may differ in the degree of competition permitted; as is the case in England and Scotland.

27  OECD, ARD Team, 'Summary of Results from Ischaemic Heart Disease Study', 2002.

28  OECD, ARD Team, 'Summary of Results from Ischaemic Heart Disease Study', 2002.

29  OECD, ARD Team, 'Summary of Results from Ischaemic Heart Disease Study', 2002.

30  OECD, ARD Team, 'Summary of Results from Ischaemic Heart Disease Study', 2002.

31  OECD, ARD Team, 'Summary of Results from Ischaemic Heart Disease Study', 2002.

32  It is unsurprising that fee-for-service payment produces higher rates of use (inappropriate supplier induced demand), however, regulation through budgets can mitigate against such behaviour.

33  OECD, ARD Team, 'Summary of Results from Ischaemic Heart Disease Study', 2002.

34  Irvine, B. and Green, D.G., *International Medical Outcomes: How does the UK compare?*, Civitas, 2003. http://www.civitas.org.uk/pdf/hpcgOutcomes.pdf Also see Appendix: http://www.civitas.org.uk/pdf/hpcgOutcomesAppendix.pdf

35  See Mossialos, E., Dixon A., Figueras, J. and Kutzin, J. (eds), *Funding Health Care: Options for Europe*, European Observatory on Health Care Systems, Buckingham: Open University Press, 2002.

36  Mossialos and Le Grand, 1999.

37  Mossialos, Dixon *et al.*, 2002.

38  The US is one obvious exception.

39  Tony Blair, speech to Fabian Society, 17 June 2003. This two-tier access to services was also emphasised in the Wanless interim report  even more recently in November 2003, the LSE Health published a report showing that access to healthcare is better for the middle classes—who know how to 'play' the system (Dixon, Le Grand, Henderson, Murray, Poteliakhoff, *Is the NHS equitable? A review of the evidence*, LSE Health and Social care Discussion Paper Number 11, 2003.

## Commentary

1  Kanavos, P., *Policy Futures for UK Health: Economy and Finance*, Technical series No. 5, London: The Nuffield Trust, 1999.

2  National Audit Office, *Measuring the Performance of Government Departments*, House of Commons Paper 301, London: The Stationery Office, 14 March 2001.

3   McKeown, T., *The Role of Medicine: dream, mirage or nemesis?*, London: Nuffield Provincial Hospitals Trust, 1976.

4   Tudor Hart, J., 'Commentary: Three decades of the inverse care law', *British Medical Journal*, 2000, 320: 18-19; Pell, J., Pell, A.C.H. *et al.*, 'Effect of socio-economic deprivation on waiting time for cardiac surgery: retrospective cohort study', *British Medical Journal*, 2000; 320: 15-17; Bunker, J., 'The role of medical care in contributing to health improvements within societies', *International Journal of Epidemiology*, (2001) 30, 1260-1263; Deaton, A. and Paxon, C., *Mortality, Income, and Income Inequality Over Time in Britain and the United States*, NBER Working Paper No. w8534, National Bureau of Economic Research, 2001.

5   Parsons, L., *Global Health: A Local Issue*, 2000. http://www.nuffieldtrust.org. uk/health2/global.intro.doc

6   National Audit Office, *International Health Comparisons*, NAO, 2003.

7   Freeman, R., *The Politics of Health in Europe*, Manchester University Press, 2000.

8   McKee, M. and Figueras, J., 'Comparing healthcare systems: how do we know if we can learn from others?', *Journal of Health Services Research and Policy*, (1997) 2(2), 122-125.

9   WHO, 2000; and WHO, 2001.

10  European Court of Justice, *Judgement of the Court, Case C-157/99*, 12 July, 2001.

11  Mossialos, E. and McKee, M., 'Is a European Healthcare Policy emerging?', *British Medical Journal*, 2001; 323, 248.

12  Woods, K., 'Health Policy and the NHS in the UK 1997-2002', in Adams, J. and Robinson, P. (eds), *Devolution in Practice*, London: The Institute of Public Policy Research (IPPR) and the ESRC, 2002.

13  Parkin, D., 'Comparing health service efficiency across countries', *Oxford Review of Economic Policy*, (1989) 5(1), 75-88; Kanavos, P. and Mossialos E., 'International comparisons of healthcare expenditures: what we know and what we do not know?', *Journal of Health Services Research and Policy*, (1999) 4(2), 122-126.

14  Williams, A., 'Science or marketing at WHO? A commentary on 'World Health 2000', *Health Economics*, (2001) 10, 93-100.

15 NHS Executive, *The NHS Performance Assessment Framework*, Department of Health, 1999; Scottish Executive Health Department, *New Performance Assessment and Accountability Review Arrangements for NHSScotland*, Edinburgh: Scottish Executive, 2001; NHS Wales, *Improving Health in Wales: A Plan for the NHS and its Partners*, Cardiff: National Assembly for Wales, 2001.

16 Mulligan, J., Appleby, J. and Harrison, A., 'Measuring the Performance of Health Systems', *British Medical Journal,*; 2000; 321, 191-192; Navarro, V., 'Assessment of the World Health Report 2000', *Lancet* (2000) 356 (4) 1598-1601; Hurst, J. and Jee-Hughes, M.,*'Performance Measurement and Performance Management in OECD Health Systems'*, Labour Market and Social Policy Occasional Papers, No. 47, OECD, January, 2001.

17 Freeman, R., *New Knowledge in New Settings: social learning in the health sector*, European Science Foundation, Standing Committee for the Social Sciences (SCSS), 2001; Freeman, R. and Woods, K.,'Learning from Devolution: UK Policy Since 1999', *British Journal of Health Care Management*, (2002) Vol 8, (12) 461-466.

18 DiMaggio, P.J. and Powell, W.W., 'The iron cage revisited: institutional isomorphism and collective rationality in organizational fields', in Powell, W.W. and DiMaggio, P.J. (eds), *The New Institutionalism in Organizational Analysis*, Chicago: University of Chicago Press, 1991; Radaelli, C., 'Policy transfer in the European Union: institutional isomorphism as a source of legitimacy', *Governance* (2000) 13 (1) 25-44.

19 OECD various; Ham, C., *'Health Care Reform: Learning from International Experience.'* Buckingham: Open University Press, 1997.

20 Bullivant, J., *'Benchmarking for Continuous Improvement in the Public Sector'*, Longman, 1994; Bullivant, J., *'Benchmarking for Best Value in the NHS'*, London: Financial Times Healthcare, 1998.

21 Parkin, 1989; Kanavos and Mossialos, 'International comparisons of healthcare expenditures', 1999.

22 Or, Z., *Exploring the Effects of Health Care on Mortality Across OECD Countries*. Labour market and social policy – Occasional Papers, No. 46, Paris: OECD, 2000; Or, Z., 'Determinants of health outcomes in industrialised countries: a pooled cross-

country, time-series analysis', *OECD Economic Studies*, Vol. 2000/1, No. 30, 2000A.

23 District Audit Wales, *'Maturity Matrices'*, January 2001.

24 Donaldson, L. J., Kirkup, W., Craig, N. and Parkin, D., 'Lanterns in the Jungle: Is the NHS Driven by the Wrong Kind of Efficiency?', *Public Health*, (1994) 108:3-9.

25 Entwistle, V.A., 'Supporting and Resourcing Treatment Decision-making: Some Policy Considerations', *Health Expectations* (2000) 3(1) 77-75.

26 E.g. Wensing, M. and Grol, R., 'What can patients do to improve health care?', *Health Expectations* (1998) 1(1) 37-49.

27 Coulter, A. and Cleary, P.D., 'Patients Experiences with hospital care in Five Countries', *Health Affairs*, (2001) 20(3) 244-252.

28 Marshall, M., Shekelle, P., Brook, P. and Leatherman, S., *Dying to Know, Public Release of Information about Quality of Health Care*, Nuffield Trust Series No. 12, Co-published with RAND, 2000.

29 Dolowitz, D. and Marsh, D., 'Who Learns What from Whom: a review of the policy transfer literature', *Political Studies* (1996) XLIV (2) 343-357; Evans, M. and Davies, J., 'Understanding policy transfer: a multi-level, multi-disciplinary perspective', *Public Administration* (1999) 77 (2) 361-385; Klein, R., 'Learning from others: shall the last be the first?' *Journal of Health Politics, Policy and Law* (1997) 22 (5) 1267-1278; Marmor, T.R., Okma, K.G.H., 'Cautionary lessons from the west: what (not) to learn from other countries' experiences in the financing and delivery of health care', in Flora, P., de Jong, P.R., Le Grand, J. and Kim, J-Y. (eds), *The State of Social Welfare, 1997*, International studies on social insurance and retirement, employment, family policy and health care, Aldershot: Ashgate, 1998.

30 Klein, R., 'Risks and benefits of comparative studies: notes from another shore', *Milbank Quarterly* (1991) 69 (2) 275-291; Bechhofer, F. and Paterson, L,. *Principles of Research Design in the Social Sciences,* London: Routledge, 2000; and Bolderson, H., Mabbett, D., Hudson, J., Rowe, M. and Spicker, P., *Delivering Social Security: A Cross-National Study*, Report of research carried out by the Department of Government at Brunel University on behalf of the Department of Social Security, London: Stationery Office, 1997.

31 Freeman, *New Knowledge in New Settings,* 2001.

32 Merton, R. and Kendall, P., 'The Focused Interview', American *Journal of Sociology* (1946) 51 (6) 541-557.

33 Feacham, R.G.A., Neelam, K.S. and White, K.L., 'Getting more for their dollar: a comparison of the NHS with California's Kaiser Permanente', *British Medical Journal*, 2002; 324, 135-143.

34 Woolhander, S., Campbell, T. and Himmelstein, D.U., 'Costs of Health Care Administration in the United States and Canada', *New England Journal of Medicine*, (2003) 349, 768-775.

35 Leon, D., Morton, S., Cannegieter, S. and McKee, M., *Understanding the Health of Scotland's Population in an International Context: A review of current approaches, knowledge and recommendations for new research directions,* Part 1, LSHTM, November 2002 (Revised).

36 Public Health Institute for Scotland, 2001, *Chasing the Scottish Effect,* PHIS, Clifton House, Glasgow. www.phis.org.uk

37 Naylor, D., Karey, I. and Handa, K., 'Measuring Health System Performance: Problems and Opportunities in an Era of Assessment and Accountability', Paper in 'Measuring up: Improving Health Systems Performance in OECD Countries' *OECD Conference*, Ottawa, 5 November, 2001.